The
Healing
Power of
Minerals,
Special Nutrients,
and Trace Elements

PAUL BERGNER

PRIMA PUBLISHING

*To Weston and Florence Price, and to Pat Connolly and the
volunteer directors of the Price-Pottenger Nutrition Foundation.*

Warning — Disclaimer
Prima Publishing has designed this book to provide information in regard to the subject matter covered. It is sold with the understanding that the publisher and the author are not liable for the misconception or misuse of information provided. Every effort has been made to make this book as complete and as accurate as possible. The author and Prima Publishing shall have neither liability nor responsibility to any person or entity with respect to any loss, damage, or injury caused or alleged to be caused directly or indirectly by the information contained in this book. The information presented herein is in no way intended as a substitute for medical counseling.

PRIMA PUBLISHING and colophon are registered trademarks of Prima Communications, Inc.

Library of Congress Cataloging-in-Publication Data
Bergner, Paul.
    The healing power of minerals, special nutrients, and trace elements /
    Paul Bergner.
        p.   cm.
    Includes bibliographical references and index.
    ISBN 0-7615-1021-4
    1. Minerals in human nutrition.   2. Trace elements in nutrition.
3. Dietary supplements.   I. Title.
QP533.B47   1997
612.3'924—dc21   97-20545
                                                                    CIP

97 98 99 00 01 HH 10 9 8 7 6 5 4 3 2 1
Printed in the United States of America

HOW TO ORDER
Single copies may be ordered from Prima Publishing, P.O. Box 1260BK, Rocklin, CA 95677; telephone (916) 632-4400. Quantity discounts are available. On your letterhead, include information concerning the intended use of the books and the number of books you wish to purchase.

Visit us online at http://www.primapublishing.com

CONTENTS

ACKNOWLEDGMENTS

The completion of this book would have been impossible without the contributions of Jonathan Merritt and Jenifer Means, N.D., L.Ac., who researched and wrote the first draft of Section 2, "Minerals in Health and Disease."

Thanks also to Sally Fallon, who steered me right on some of the fine points of Weston Price's research, to the Price-Pottenger Nutrition Foundation and Keats Publishing for permission to reprint photographs from *Nutrition and Physical Degeneration* by Weston Price, and to Ryan Drum, Ph.D., for world-class information on sea vegetables.

I also used *The Kellogg Report: the Impact of Nutrition, Environment, and Lifestyle on the Health of Americans* by Dr. Joseph Beasley as a primary resource for background information.

Finally, thanks to Bill Vail for productive discussions of the material and for his encouragement and support.

INTRODUCTION

The European alchemists of the Middle Ages worked and experimented extensively with minerals. They strove to complete the "Great Work"—to turn lead into gold. The alchemists' labors consisted of acquiring minerals—many more than just lead and gold—purifying them chemically, and combining them in various ways in an effort to discover the science of their transformation. Alchemy is portrayed as ignorance today in basic chemistry texts, but it ultimately gave birth to the modern sciences of chemistry and nuclear physics.

ALCHEMY IN NATURE AND NUTRITION

A close look at the universe, geology, biology, and human nutrition shows that alchemical transformation of minerals not only occurs, it is the hidden secret behind the way nature works. In the radioactive turmoil of the sun, hydrogen is transmuted into all the natural elements in the universe—seventy-five of them minerals. The process continues in the hot magma deep in the earth, and the minerals rise to be diffused throughout the earth's crust and dissolved in the sea in the form of salts. Sea plants selectively assimilate minerals and concentrate them in the balance and proportions necessary for the food of animals.

In the earth's crust and soil, bacteria and other microorganisms ingest and transform the minerals into a form suitable for land plants to use. The plants assimilate them so they're suitable for animals. Animals, including humans, eat the plants or other animals. You will see in Chapters 2 and 27 that a diet rich in *both* plant and animal foods provides optimum nutrition for the human being. In the human body, minerals act as catalysts, participating in enzyme systems that allow the transformation of the food and air we breathe into energy, vibrant health, and consciousness. In Chapters 5 to 24, I'll describe the role of each of twenty-two minerals in health and disease, and how they interact with vitamins and other nutrients.

ALCHEMY GONE AWRY

Traditional farmer-alchemists throughout the history of agriculture have been careful to return their mineral-rich plant and animal wastes to the soil, thus preserving the minerals and making them available to the soil bacteria and plants. Traditional people, as we'll see in Chapter 2, often went to great lengths to obtain mineral-rich foods, and consumed only natural, whole foods. In Chapters 2 and 3, you'll see how modern food processing and agricultural methods strip the soil and our food of their mineral content, reducing mineral availability to the "alchemist's workshop" of our bodies. In Chapters 2, 4, and 25, I'll illustrate the result of the modern diet on the mineral status of Americans.

Modern medicine, although it documents their deficiencies in the population, generally ignores minerals' significance and employs powerful but inappropriate drugs to treat disease, instead of first respecting the natural alchemy of minerals and health and restoring the optimal mineral nutrition of the body. The secret work of the alchemists of the Middle Ages was to turn the lead of the human character into the gold of spirituality. We'll see in Chapter 25 that if the minerals in our body become deficient, we experience fatigue, irritability, depression, and anxiety, and our immune system begins to lose its control over biological invaders. We end up less able to perform our spiritual work, whether it is service to our families, communities, nature, humanity, or the Creator.

ALCHEMY AND THE DIET

The alchemist sometimes had to go to great lengths to acquire his metals and the knowledge of how to use them. Today, we have to extend effort, and sometimes money, to seek out and acquire the mineral-rich foods our bodies need. We may also have to spend time cooking them, rather than eating fast food. In Chapters 26 to 29, you will learn how to obtain your minerals from food available today—despite the general demineralization of agricultural products and the standard American diet—and assimilate them into your body. If we respect the pattern of the alchemy of minerals in nature, and consume mineral-rich foods in their natural forms, our health will improve. We can then go about our Great Work with more vigor, energy, mental clarity, and peace.

From the Earth to Your Body

All flesh is grass.

Isaiah 40:6

NINETY-TWO elements occur in nature, all derived from nuclear reactions that take place within the sun or deep within the earth. Thirteen elements have no important role in the biological functioning of living things—seven of these are radioactive and six are inert gasses. Four elements—carbon, hydrogen, oxygen, and nitrogen—are the basic building blocks of organic life. The remaining seventy-five elements are classified as minerals. Their role in health and disease is the subject of this book.

Scientists have either proven or suggested a beneficial role in animal life for thirty-one minerals (see the box "Thirty-One Minerals Beneficial to Animal Life"). The other forty-four minerals may or may not play a role in health and disease. For the most part, they have not been investigated. They exist in living things in such a small concentration—parts per million or parts per billion—that analytical equipment has only been available to measure their presence for a few decades. Despite the minute concentrations, some of the minerals listed following have important biological functions. There is little doubt that the

1

importance of many more of these minerals will eventually be identified. Most of them exist in the natural environment of the sea, where life arose, and also are present in the rocks and soils of the earth. Based on their prevalence on the planet, it seems reasonable to propose that some of them may play subtle and important roles in sustaining animal life.

As a class of nutrients, minerals have three major roles in the body: They provide structural materials for the bones and other connective tissues; they allow electrical impulses to move along the nerves; and they act as catalysts or support the role of enzymes in physiological processes, such as replication of DNA or manufacture of proteins. Catalysts and enzymes promote the transformation of one thing into another. The spark plugs in your car act as catalysts when they initiate the transformation of gasoline into energy. Your digestive enzymes promote the transformation of the food you eat into components that can be absorbed in the intestine. The vital role minerals play accounts for the devastating effects of certain mineral deficiencies on our health. Magnesium participates in more than one hundred enzymatic reactions in the body, and zinc in more than two hundred. A deficiency of these two minerals alone can result in three hundred different health problems. Without the proper minerals, you are like a car running without all its spark plugs.

In nutrition, minerals are conventionally categorized as major minerals or trace elements. The arbitrary marker of a major mineral is one having a daily requirement of more than 100 milligrams. Note that this dose is at the level of parts per million for a 150-pound adult. The major minerals are:

calcium
chlorine
magnesium
phosphorus

potassium
sodium
sulfur

All other minerals listed in the box "Thirty-One Minerals Beneficial to Animal Life" are classified as trace elements. Some of these trace elements are active in the body in daily doses in the range of micrograms (1 microgram is 0.01 milligram), which falls in the range of parts per billion by weight for an adult human. Perhaps the most well-known trace element is iron, which was first discovered in the seventeenth century to be essential to health. It is added to many of our processed foods today to ensure that we do not develop deficiencies. Iodine is another well-known mineral. In the nineteenth century researchers discovered that iodine supplements can cure or prevent goiter.

THIRTY-ONE MINERALS BENEFICIAL TO ANIMAL LIFE*

Aluminum	Fluorine	Phosphorus
Arsenic	Gallium	Potassium
Barium	Germanium	Selenium
Boron	Iodine	Silicon
Bromine	Iron	Sodium
Cadmium	Lead	Sulfur
Calcium	Lithium	Tin
Chlorine	Magnesium	Vanadium
Chromium	Manganese	Zinc
Cobalt	Molybdenum	
Copper	Nickel	

*Several of these are beneficial in tiny doses, but poisonous in larger doses.

Since then, iodine has been added to table salt to ensure that the American public receives a minimum dose.

Some minerals that are essential in tiny doses are extremely poisonous in larger doses. For centuries they have been the subject of crime stories, political intrigue, and occupational tragedies in Western civilization. Lead in the water supply has even been proposed as the cause of the fall of the Roman empire. The most toxic minerals are listed here. Mercury is the only one listed that is not beneficial even in tiny doses.

aluminum
arsenic
cadmium
lead
mercury

Most minerals, even calcium, can be toxic if you take too much, something to remember when taking them as supplements. I discuss supplements in great detail in Section 3, "Getting the Minerals You Need."

In Section 1 you'll learn how minerals make the journey from the volcanic rock of the earth or the dissolved minerals of the sea to your body. I'll explain how ancient people following a traditional diet usually did not suffer from mineral deficiencies. You will see how the food chain is disrupted by unwise agricultural techniques, how the food we eat has become radically demineralized in the last century, and better understand the impact of demineralization on public health.

CHAPTER 1

FROM THE COSMOS TO YOUR TABLE

We created man from mud, molded into shape.

Quran 15:26

Whether we accept the revelations of the scriptures or the theories of evolutionary scientists, we reach the same conclusion: The human body is molded from the elements of water and earth, from the materials in the earth's crust, and from the elements in the water of the oceans, mixed together like mud or clay. Most of the ninety-two naturally occurring elements of the earth also exist in the human body, and most of the dissolved mineral elements of the sea occur naturally in the fluids of the human body. The combination of these elements is essential to life.

The healthy human body is a microcosm of the earth: a physical body composed of the elements of the earth and atmosphere, carrying within it an inner "sea." Regular intake of many of these earthly elements is necessary to maintain health and prevent disease. In this chapter, I'll show how the earth's and sea's minerals were formed, and how they rise through the food chain to become contained in the food on your table.

From Sun to Earth

The earth was born from the sun. Scientists do not agree on all the finer points, but the sun spun off parts of itself, either as eruptions from within or as clouds of hot, radioactive gasses. This material cooled to form the planets. During the cooling process, the radioactive elements of the sun formed new elements—ninety-two in all have been identified, including the original components of the sun.

Hydrogen Building Blocks

The sun's heat and radiation are generated by a massive, ongoing nuclear hydrogen explosion. The hydrogen atom of the sun and other stars is the basic building block of all the elements in the universe—minerals, gasses, and radioactive elements, for example—its atom contains one proton and one electron. If we could freeze it in time, it would look like a tiny moon revolving around a much larger planet. All the other elements are made from hydrogen protons and electrons reacting in the intense nuclear heat of stars; in the scattering and cooling of elements when a star explodes in a supernova; as it spins off gasses or parts of itself that cool and become planets; or in ongoing nuclear reactions deep within the planets.

Six hydrogen atoms combine to make up a carbon atom. Eleven hydrogen atoms make up the sodium in table salt. Twelve make up magnesium, nineteen potassium, twenty calcium, and ninety-two make up uranium. Besides the ninety-two minerals known to occur naturally on earth, another thirteen have been created in nuclear reactors. Some of these live very short lives—only tiny fractions of a second—before they degrade into other elements.

THE COOLING OF THE EARTH INTO LAYERS

After the initial eruption, the earth cooled to become a revolving globe of hot, liquid, radioactive material. As elements formed through ongoing nuclear fusion (the joining of existing elements) or fission (the splitting of elements), the heavier ones sank toward the core of the earth and the lighter ones rose toward the surface. As the earth continued to cool, hydrogen and oxygen formed the water of the oceans, and nitrogen, oxygen, and other gasses rose to create the atmosphere. Today, we divide the earth and its environment into seven layers: From the center moving outward, there is a solid inner core, a molten outer core, a semisolid mantle, a thin dough-like layer called the Moho, a dry crust, the sea, and the atmosphere—all created from the original radioactive matter of the sun. Table 1.1 shows the size and state of the different layers of the earth.

The Earth's Layers

The earth continues to evolve geologically. The center of activity for this evolution is in the mantle, composed of semisolid radioactive rock. Within the mantle are nuclear hot spots

TABLE 1.1   THE LAYERS OF THE EARTH

Layer	State	Depth
Inner core	solid	800 miles
Outer core	molten	1,350 miles
Mantle	semisolid	1,685 miles
Moho	dough-like	100 miles
Crust	solid	25 miles
Sea	liquid	2.5 miles
Atmosphere	gas	up to 13,000 miles

that geologists call *heaters*. These heaters act as nuclear reactors, continually generating elements through the fusion of lighter atoms in the same process that generated the layers of the earth. Due to the intense gravitational pressures of the earth above the mantle, the radioactive elements sometimes reach critical mass, causing a nuclear fission explosion—the same sequence of events that occurs when a nuclear bomb detonates. The explosion blows some material upward and downward; the upward force causes the rising and shifting of the land masses on the earth's crust. When the force of these explosions breaks through the earth's crust, we witness the eruption of a volcano. The upward thrusts also scatter all the elements above the mantle toward the crust.

Geologists believe that at one point in the evolution of the planet, volcanic activity predominated, with constant volcanic explosions spreading mineral-laden debris across the earth and into the atmosphere. The dust from a major volcanic explosion today can affect weather patterns the world over. Imagine the density of the dust-mineral cloud at a time when volcanoes dominated the earth's surface. The mixing of the upthrust rocks and the settling volcanic debris covered the continents and the ocean floor with a well-balanced mixture of all the minerals and other elements essential to life.

The Moho layer—short for the Mohorovicic discontinuity—is significant because of its consistency. Think of it as something like bread dough, with the hot, gooey, radioactive thinner batter of the mantle beneath it and the dried crust of the earth on top. The constant movement of the crust's continents, which is much too slow for us to perceive, occurs across this doughy layer of matter beneath them.

The sea contains within it, in solution, most of the minerals contained in the crust beneath it; the volcanic dust that has settled in it; and materials washed into it by rivers. Life arose in the sea, probably on its floor near the volcanic vents of the heaters in the mantle.

FROM EARTH TO SEA: THE BEGINNING OF LIFE

Picture the earth before the continents arose. The globe is covered with a vast ocean whose waters were much like today's seawater—salty. Yet the ocean has always contained much more than the sodium and chloride of common table salt. Seawater holds sixty-five minerals, all floating in solution (see Table 1.2 and Boxes 1.1 and 1.2). Deep under the sea, near the hot volcanic vents on the ocean floor, the first living molecules formed—proteins capable of reproducing themselves. These proteins were the precursors of the deoxyribonucleic acid (DNA) and ribonucleic acid (RNA) in the nucleus of living cells, which permit those cells to reproduce and carry on their metabolic functions. Scientists believe that the formation of these proteins required both the heat of the volcanic ocean floor and the minerals in the water. DNA and RNA still require these same minerals to reproduce.

THE "MINERAL HUNGER" OF LIVING CELLS

Eventually living cells evolved, wrapping the original molecules of life in a membrane. The membrane forms a barrier that allows the cell to take in certain nutrients and minerals selectively and concentrate them, creating an inner environment more favorable to the nuclear proteins. The intracellular environment of a single-celled sea plant or animal contains most of the elements of the sea itself, but in very different concentrations.

TABLE 1.2   MINERAL ELEMENTS IN SEAWATER

Mineral	Parts per Million	Mineral	Parts per Million
aluminum	0.01	magnesium	1,350.0
antimony	0.00033	manganese	0.002
arsenic	0.003	mercury	0.00003
barium	0.03	molybdenum	0.01
beryllium	0.0000006	nickel	0.0054
bismuth	0.000017	niobium	0.00001
boron	4.6	phosphorus	0.07
bromine	65.0	potassium	0.380
cadmium	0.00011	rubidium	0.12
calcium	400.0	scandium	0.000004
cerium	0.0004	selenium	0.00009
cesium	0.0005	silicon	3.0
chlorine	19,000.0	silver	0.0003
chromium	0.00005	sodium	10,500.0
cobalt	0.00027	strontium	8.1
copper	0.003	sulfur	885.0
fluorine	1.3	tantalum	0.0000025
gallium	0.00003	thallium	0.00001
germanium	0.00007	thorium	0.00005
gold	0.000011	tin	0.003
hafnium	0.000008	titanium	0.001
iodine	0.06	tungsten	0.0001
iron	0.01	vanadium	0.002
lanthanum	0.000012	yttrium	0.0003
lead	0.00003	zinc	0.01
lithium	0.18	zirconium	0.000022

Table 1.3 shows how the cells of sea plants concentrate the minerals of the sea, in some cases more than a million times. This table dramatically demonstrates the mineral hunger of living cells. Some of these minerals seem to increase the efficiency of DNA and RNA reproduction in the nuclei of plant cells.

Box 1.1
How Small Is a Part per Million?

The standard measure of mineral content in rock, water, plants, animals, and human beings is in *parts per million,* the measure used in the tables in this chapter. The number *one million* is too large for most of us to conceive, so here's some simple math to help put it into perspective. Assume a pinch of salt—sodium chloride—is about the size of a drop of water. Sixteen drops make 1 milliliter; 30 milliliters make about 1 ounce; 32 ounces make 1 quart; and 4 quarts make 1 gallon. So a gallon contains a little more than 61,000 drops of water, and a single drop would be 1 part per million in about 16 gallons of water.

Our pinch of salt is only about a half-pinch each of sodium and chloride, however, so to get 1 part per million of each, we'd have to put that pinch into about 32 gallons of water. This may seem insignificantly small, but some minerals at such concentrations in plants, animals, and humans are absolutely essential to life. Chromium, cobalt, manganese, molybdenum, and nickel—all essential to human life—are found in the body in concentrations of less than 1 part per million. Some of the minerals in Table 1.2—those with more than three zeroes after the decimal point—are measures in parts per *billion.* It would take 32,000 gallons of water to hold a concentration of 1 part per billion of our pinch of salt.

Minerals in the Food Chain of the Sea

The phrase "Big fish eat little fish, little fish eat worms, and worms eat mud" is not accurate. In fact, big fish eat little fish, little fish eat sea plants, and sea plants eat minerals and other

BOX 1.2
OTHER MINERALS IN THE SEA

Seawater has not been tested in published research for a number of trace elements. The following minerals do not appear in Table 1.2, but because they have been identified in sea plants and animals, we can assume they are also in the seawater.

Erbium	Praseodymium
Europium	Rhenium
Gadolinium	Samarium
Holmium	Tellurium
Lutetium	Terbium
Neodymium	Ytterbium

substances from the sea. Near the bottom of the food chain, the smallest fish and animals eat small single- or multicelled plants such as algae or plankton. At the top of the chain, seals, whales, other sea mammals, and humans eat big fish. Table 1.4 shows how these minerals move up the food chain and concentrate in sea animals. Animals usually have lower mineral-concentration levels than those of plants. Nevertheless, the concentration in the animals generally remains many times that found in seawater. Sea plants and animals are among the best food sources of minerals and trace elements (see Chapter 30).

THE INNER SEA OF LAND ANIMALS

When life emerged from the sea onto dry land, it did not leave the sea behind. The land animals then—and all animals today, including human beings—carry a replica of that original sea

TABLE 1.3 HOW SEA PLANTS CONCENTRATE SEA MINERALS

Mineral	Seawater (ppm)	Sea Plants (avg. ppm)	Concentration (times)
arsenic	0.003	30.0	10,000
barium	0.03	30.0	1,000
beryllium	0.0000006	0.001	1,670
bromine	65.0	740.0	11
cadmium	0.00011	0.04	363
calcium	400.0	145,000.0	362
cesium	0.00005	0.07	1,400
chromium	0.00005	1.0	20,000
cobalt	0.00027	0.7	2,592
copper	0.0003	11.0	36,666
fluorine	1.3	4.5	3
gallium	0.00005	0.5	16,666
gold	0.000011	0.01	909
hafnium	0.0000008	0.4	500,000
iodine	0.06	735.0	12,250
iron	0.01	700.0	70,000
lanthanum	0.0000012	10.0	8,333,333
lead	0.00003	8.4	280,000
lithium	0.18	5.0	27
magnesium	1,350.0	5,200.0	4
manganese	0.0002	29.0	145,000
mercury	0.00003	0.03	1,000
molybdenum	0.01	0.45	45
nickel	0.0054	3.0	555
phosphorus	0.07	3,500.0	50,000
potassium	380.0	52,000.0	136
rubidium	0.12	7.4	61
selenium	0.00009	0.8	8,888
silicon	3.0	9,250.0	3,083
silver	0.00003	0.25	8,333
sodium	10,500.0	33,000.0	3
strontium	8.1	570.0	70
sulfur	885.0	12,000.0	13
thorium	0.00005	0.0	200
tin	0.003	1.0	333
titanium	0.001	33.0	33,000
vanadium	0.002	2.0	1,000
zinc	0.01	150.0	15,000
zirconium	0.0000022	20.0	909,090

TABLE 1.4   SOME MINERALS IN THE
FOOD CHAIN OF THE SEA

Mineral*	Seawater	Sea Plants	Sea Animals
barium	0.03	30.00	2.50
bromine	65.00	740.00	470.00
calcium	400.00	145,000.00	9,250.00
fluorine	1.30	4.50	2.00
iodine	0.06	735.00	75.00
iron	0.01	700.00	400.00
lanthanum	0.00	10.00	0.01
lithium	0.18	5.00	1.00
magnesium	1,350.00	5,200.00	5,000.00
molybdenum	0.01	0.45	1.25
nickel	0.01	3.00	12.70
phosphorus	0.07	3,500.00	7,000.00
potassium	380.00	2,000.00	12,500.00
rubidium	0.12	7.40	20.00
silicon	3.00	9,250.00	70,000.00
sodium	10,500.00	33,000.00	22,000.00
strontium	8.10	570.00	260.00
sulfur	885.00	12,000.00	7,000.00
zinc	0.01	150.00	753.00

*Concentrations in parts per million

within us in the *extracellular fluid,* that one-fifth of our body fluids that bathes and nourishes every cell in our body. This fluid
has a similar mineral composition to the original sea from which
life emerged. The body strictly maintains the mineral content of
the fluid to resemble that of the prehistoric sea—even robbing
minerals from the bones or other tissue to do so. When the
body steals minerals from tissues to maintain a steady balance
in the body fluids, pathology arises in the form of one of many
mineral-deficiency diseases like osteoporosis. Table 1.5 compares the concentration of minerals in the nuclei of human cells

TABLE 1.5   MINERALS IN SEA PLANTS
             AND HUMAN CELLS

Mineral*	Sea Plants	Human Cell Nuclei
calcium	145,000	13,500
cobalt	0.7	0.46
copper	11	7
iron	700	140
potassium	52,000	20,400
magnesium	5,200	800
manganese	29	1–17
sodium	33,000	6,300
phosphorus	3,500	25,000
sulfur	12,000	1,500
zinc	150	3–140

*Concentrations in parts per million

with the concentration in sea plants. Notice that the figures, while not identical, are all of the same order of magnitude. The sea plant's habit of concentrating certain minerals from the sea (see Table 1.3) set the precedent for all future life. These levels remain essential for cell function and reproduction.

THE FOOD CHAIN OF LAND ANIMALS

Unlike sea plants, humans and other land animals cannot draw their minerals directly from the sea. Seawater, if drunk in sufficient quantities to provide enough minerals, will kill a human being. The mineral composition of our body fluids depends entirely on our diet. Unless we eat seafood, our minerals must be taken from the earth's crust.

Of course you cannot eat a piece of granite or other volcanic rock — it must first be transformed into soil. The land food chain follows five stages.

Stage 1

Volcanic activity from the magma of the earth forms volcanic rock, either thrust upward violently in volcanoes or pushed up less dramatically during the upthrusting of the earth's crust. All but two of the mineral elements have been found at measurable levels in volcanic rock (see Table 1.6).

Stage 2

Weather, geological, oceanic, or bacterial activity continually breaks rock into smaller pieces and particles, even crushing it into dust. Plants and their roots can also break up rock, as you can see when grass breaks down a cement sidewalk. Life formed more easily in the sea, but, once formed, it had no problem penetrating to the earth's crust. Geologists have found bacteria and other microorganisms at depths thousands of feet below the crust. These also break down and degrade rock. Some rock, such as limestone, is formed when minerals from the sea collect to form the rock. Limestone and other such rock is dispersed all over the earth, which was once entirely under water.

Stage 3

Bacteria and other soil organisms assimilate minerals from the rock. When the organisms die, the minerals are dispersed in the soil. This stage, which I will discuss in detail in Chapter 4, is absolutely essential to all life on earth, because it provides food for plant roots in a usable form. If the bacteria and other organisms in the soil die, the soil itself is dead as far as plant life is concerned; the plants starve for lack of nutrients. Table 1.7 shows the result of the bacterial ingestion of rock on the soil content of minerals.

TABLE 1.6   THE MINERAL CONTENT
OF VOLCANIC ROCK

Mineral	Parts per Million	Mineral	Parts per Million
aluminum	5,000	molybdenum	1.5
antimony	0.2	neodymium	28
arsenic	1–8	nickel	75
barium	425	osmium	0.0015
beryllium	2–8	palladium	0.01
bismuth	0.17	phosphorus	1,050
boron	10	platinum	0.005
bromine	3–5	polonium	2–10
cadmium	0.2	potassium	20,000
calcium	41,500	praseodymium	8.2
cerium	60	rhenium	0.005
cesium	1	rhodium	0.001
chlorine	130	rubidium	90
chromium	100	ruthenium	0.001
cobalt	25	samarium	6
copper	55	scandium	22
dysprosium	3	selenium	0.05
erbium	2.8	silicon	281,500
europium	1–3	silver	0.07
fluorine	625	sodium	23,600
gadolinium	5.4	strontium	375
gallium	15	sulfur	260
germanium	5.4	tantalum	2
hafnium	3	tellurium	0.001
holmium	1.2	terbium	0.9
indium	0.05–1	thallium	0.45
iodine	0.5	thorium	6–9
iridium	0.001	thulium	0.48
iron	56,300	tin	2
lanthanum	30	titanium	5,700
lead	2.5	tungsten	1.5
lithium	20	vanadium	135
lutetium	0.5	ytterbium	3
magnesium	23,000	yttrium	33
manganese	950	zinc	70
mercury	0.08	zirconium	165

TABLE 1.7   THE MINERAL CONTENT
OF ROCK AND SOIL

Mineral*	Volcanic Rock	Soil
bromine	3–5	2–100
calcium	41,500	5
chlorine	130	4,000–50,000
chromium	100	100
copper	55	5–3,000
fluorine	625	2–100
gallium	15	0.4–6
lithium	20	30
magnesium	23,000	5,000
molybdenum	1.5	2
nickel	75	40
potassium	20,000	14,000
sodium	23,600	6,300
sulfur	260	700
tin	2	2–200
zinc	70	50

*Concentrations in parts per million

Stage 4

Plants assimilate minerals from the soil. A plant's "intestines" are its roots. The tiny root hairs closely resemble the tiny protrusions in your intestines that allow your body to assimilate the food you eat. Minerals are dispersed throughout every part of the plant, some of them more concentrated in certain areas. As plants die, they decompose and leave their minerals on the surface of the soil, enriching the surface soil layer. Plants with deep roots tap into minerals from deep within the earth, and, when decomposing, deposit them on the surface, providing mineral food for smaller plants with shorter roots.

Breaking this cycle by harvesting and carrying away the plants eventually causes demineralization of the soil and a loss of fertility, which I discuss at length in Chapter 4.

Stage 5

Animals—humans included—eat plants. For many animals, plants provide the only food source of minerals. Elephants, which are herbivores, acquire from plant sources all the calcium they need to support their immense bones and tusks.

COMPARING THE FOOD CHAINS OF THE LAND AND SEA

Table 1.8 shows the movement of twenty essential minerals through the food chain from rock through soil and into plants and animals. Compare the movement to that of the food chain of the sea (Table 1.4). In the sea, plants and animals greatly concentrate minerals. The opposite is true in the land food chain. The concentrations of most of the minerals gradually decline as they move up the chain. In the sea, we start the chain with tiny amounts of minerals in the water. On land, we start with a great abundance of minerals in the earth's crust. The soil microorganisms take what they need and leave the rest, and so on up the chain.

This land food chain is much more fragile than that of the sea. Sea plants can absorb their minerals directly from an inexhaustible supply—seawater. On land, however, the transformation of rock to soil is an extra link in the chain. To maintain an unbroken chain on the land, soil microorganisms must thrive, and the minerals in decomposing plants must be recycled into the soil. Modern industrial agriculture skips this important step. Crops are not rotated, fertilizers only contain a handful of

TABLE 1.8   ESSENTIAL MINERALS IN THE
FOOD CHAIN OF THE LAND

Mineral*	Rock	Soil	Plants	Animals
arsenic	1–8	6	0.2	0.2
bromine	3–5	5	15	6
cadmium	0.2	0.06	0.06	0.5
calcium	41,500	4,000–50,000	18,000	200–85,000
chlorine	130	100	2,000	2,800
chromium	100	5–3,000	0.23	0.075
copper	55	2–100	14	2–4
fluorine	625	200	5–40	150–500
iodine	0.5	5	0.42	0.43
lead	12.5	10	2.7	2
lithium	20	30	1	0.02
magnesium	23,000	5,000	3,200	1,000
molybdenum	1.5	2	0.9	0.2
nickel	75	40	3	0.08
potassium	20,000	14,000	14,000	7,400
sodium	23,600	6,300	1,200	4,000
sulfur	260	700	3,400	5,000
tin	2	2–200	0.3	0.15
zinc	70	50	100	160

*Concentrations in parts per million

essential minerals, and pesticides disrupt and destroy the ecology of soil organisms. Chapter 4 focuses on this unwise practice of breaking the mineral food chain and its consequences on the mineral content of your food.

THE FINAL LINK IN THE CHAIN

The final link in the chain, as far as humans are concerned, is the dinner table. Nature has provided abundant mineral-rich foods for us to eat—more than enough to provide robust health.

Unfortunately, modern food processing removes much of the mineral content of our food, which I will discuss in greater depth in Section 3, "Getting the Minerals You Need."

Looking back at Table 1.8, notice that, in most cases, the content of minerals is higher in plants than in animals. This high mineral content in whole plants is one of the best arguments for eating a diet rich in plant foods, and contributes to the therapeutic value of such dietary practices as vegetarianism and juicing. Notice also, however, that some minerals, such as zinc, appear in much higher concentrations in animals. People who eat plant foods exclusively, unless they eat carefully and consciously, risk developing several mineral deficiencies. I'll go into more detail about this in Chapter 27.

In the next chapter you will see how traditional people who eat both plants and animals in their naturally occurring forms generally enjoy robust health almost unheard of in modern society.

CHAPTER 2

TRADITIONAL VERSUS MODERN FOODS

Life in all its fullness is Mother Nature obeyed.

Weston Price, 1938

In the last chapter I described how minerals move up the food chain from the earth and sea to the foods you eat. Nature delivers us mineral-rich foods, infused with the mineral content, vitamins, fiber, and essential fats that our bodies and spirits need to thrive. In our society, illnesses—especially low-grade mineral-deficiency diseases—are so common that we've lost sight of what true health is. In this chapter I'll describe the health of traditional peoples eating their natural diets, and show what happens to them when they start eating the modern foods that we now think of as natural.

A LANDMARK IN NUTRITION RESEARCH

The most significant nutrition book of this century, which clarifies many questions on diet and health, is *Nutrition and Physical Degeneration* by Weston Price. This book is a recommended text for my nutrition students at the Rocky Mountain Center for Botanical Studies in Boulder, Colorado. I lecture from it and use it to teach my students how to review diets and how to recommend dietary changes for clients. I recommend that you get a copy to read solid evidence of how a whole-foods natural diet—including meat—can improve your health. Price, a dentist, and his wife, Florence, traveled the world in the 1930s, visiting more than fourteen cultures from the South Pacific Islands to Africa, Switzerland, and the Outer Hebrides Islands off the coast of Scotland. In that decade the people of these cultures were in transition from their traditional diets to the foods of modern civilization. Price and his wife examined and compared the teeth and bone structure of individuals eating each kind of diet and recorded the findings with extensive photographic evidence. While their focus was on dental and bone health, they also noted the general physical and mental health of the people and commented on the types of diseases that began to appear when the modern diet was adopted.

Nutrition and Physical Degeneration was first published in 1938, and reprinted in 1970 and 1989. How many other nutrition books from that era would you imagine are still in print? The Prices' work has become more rather than less important as time passes, because the health of our nation today proves their findings and concepts to be correct. The Prices are in a historical position similar to that of Sir James Lind, who proved that citrus fruits would prevent or cure scurvy in 1753. Only in 1795, after some 100,000 British sailors had died of scurvy in forty-two years, did the British navy begin to provide its sailors with citrus fruits. Similarly, the Prices demonstrated the cause and suggested the cure for many degenerative diseases. We are now like those British sailors who died of scurvy, waiting for public policy to catch up with scientific facts.

WESTON AND FLORENCE PRICE

Weston Price was born in 1870 in southern Ontario, Canada, and was raised on a traditional farm. He earned undergraduate and dentistry degrees from the University of Michigan in Ann Arbor and set up a practice in Grand Forks, North Dakota. Shortly thereafter he developed typhoid fever and nearly died. To help him recover, Price's brother-in-law took him to a wilderness lake in Ontario, where they camped and fished, eating fish, small game, wild foods, and whatever else they brought along, until Price returned to robust health. These two experiences—growing up on a farm and recovering from a serious illness in a natural setting while eating natural foods—certainly formed in Price the basis for the insights of his later work. Price loved the lakeside setting so much that when he married Florence they honeymooned there, even though it required a twenty-mile wagon ride and a six-mile boat trip across the lake.

After his recovery, Price set up a dental practice in Cleveland. There he became passionately interested in the cause of the dental problems he saw every day. He theorized that the cause of tooth and gum problems was not a lack of hygiene but some factor in the diet. He also noted the general decline in the health of the population around him, with the city-born children he saw being in poorer health, both physically and mentally, than the mostly farm-raised adults. In 1914 he published a report on growth defects in the teeth of young children (Price, 1914). Ten years later he published a two-volume work on dental infections (Price, 1924). In his study of infection, he theorized that dietary or other factors were responsible in most cases:

The evidence seemed to indicate clearly that the forces that were at work were not to be found in the diseased tissues, but that the undesirable conditions were the result of the absence of something, rather than the presence of something. (Price, 1938)

Being of a scientific disposition, Price wanted to find a control group of individuals in good dental health so he could compare them with unhealthy individuals and uncover what difference, if any, was present in their diet and lifestyle. Unable to find large groups of healthy people in his area, he began searching the world for such societies. In his own words:

I determined to search out primitive racial stocks that were free from the degenerative process with which we are concerned in order to note what they have that we do not have. (Price, 1938)

THE PRICES' TRAVELS

Starting in 1931, Weston and Florence Price traveled the world to fourteen different regions, examining the health of indigenous people. They met and studied traditional Swiss, Gaelics of the Outer Hebrides Islands, Eskimos, North American Indians, Melanesians, Polynesians, East African tribes, Australian aborigines, New Zealand Maori, Peruvian Indians, and Amazon Indians, sometimes studying more than one group in each region. They found these societies in transition, with some villages or societies consuming a traditional diet and others nearby eating modern-day processed foods such as granulated sugar, white flour, and canned foods. Price found the ideal conditions for the experiments he sought to undertake—closely related groups who shared the same racial background but ate different diets. The Prices had to travel by airplane (no joy ride in 1938), boat, wagon, or by foot on trails to reach these people. Florence Price's contributions to the work were substantial. She accompanied Weston on the travels, and he ultimately dedicated the resulting book to her because she "assisted me so greatly on these difficult expeditions."

PRICE'S FINDINGS

What started as a quest to examine dental health ultimately revealed information about the overall health of the Prices' research subjects. Weston Price interviewed doctors and staff of hospitals near the people he studied and found that tuberculosis, arthritis, gall bladder disease, and conditions requiring surgery were rare among people eating a traditional diet, but common among those consuming the modern foods. It is difficult to describe how dramatic Price's findings were without viewing the many photographs in his book—134 black-and-white photographs showing the effects of the two diets on dental health and bone structure (see Figures 2.1, 2.2, and 2.3).

Typically, the photos first show a group of people on the traditional diet: They look in perfect dental health and have broad dental arches (no need for an orthodontist), vibrant overall health, and a peaceful or joyous look on their faces. Photos of people from the same racial background who ate modern, processed foods show missing teeth, narrow pinched faces, narrow jaws with crowded teeth, and anguished expressions.

I was struck with shock and near horror after viewing the photos and then walking out among the public in Boulder. We are a society of the people from the "after" photos, only we have had our teeth "fixed." The same deficient bony structure and pinched, pained facial expressions as those of the indigenous people eating a modern diet show everywhere on the streets of modern-day America. The night after I read Price's book, I noticed that in my class of clinical herbalists—ten women of ages running from the mid-twenties to the mid-forties—only one woman had the face and bone structure of the healthy primitive

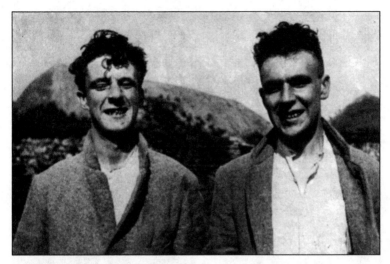

FIGURE 2.1   Brothers, Isle of Harris. The younger at left used modern food and had rampant tooth decay. Brother at right used native food and had excellent teeth. Note narrowed face and arch of younger brother. (Photo and caption reprinted from Price, 1938.)

people. She was raised in a chiropractor's family, ate whole foods, and was not allowed to eat sugar.

The photos in Price's book also reminded me of a boy in whose house I lived in the 1980s. His mother ate only organic whole foods while she was pregnant with him, raised him on the same foods, and never allowed him to eat sugar. I watched him once at age five score four goals in a soccer game with other five-year-olds. He was so robust, and they were so run-down looking, that he looked like Superman among a group of weaklings — much like the before and after pictures in Price's book. My casual observations supported one of Price's key points: Diet during pregnancy and childhood can determine the state of health in adult life, even if an individual begins to eat poorly later on. He found the practice of preparing a mother for pregnancy

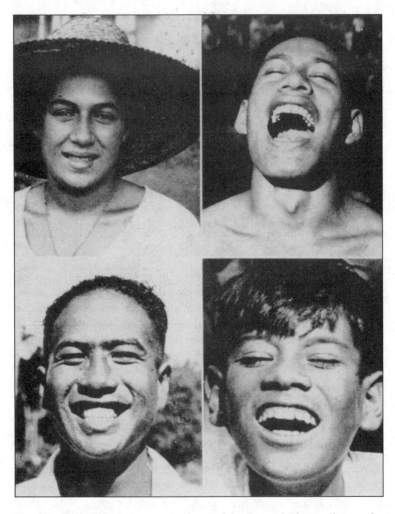

FIGURE 2.2 Polynesians are a beautiful race and physically sturdy. They have straight hair and their color is often that of a suntanned European. They have perfect dental arches. (Photos and caption reprinted from Price, 1938.)

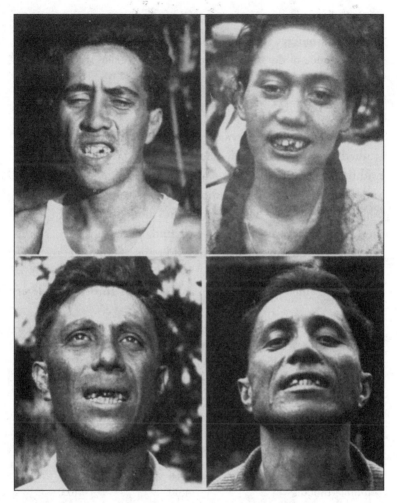

FIGURE 2.3 Where the native foods have been displaced by the imported foods, dental caries become rampant. These are typical modernized Tahitians. (Photos and caption reprinted from Price, 1938.)

by feeding her special, nutrient-rich foods to be widespread among the indigenous cultures. Table 2.1 shows the comparative incidence of dental caries in the groups Price studied.

THE TRADITIONAL DIETS

The Prices found a wide variety of diets among the people they studied (see Table 2.2). The most common differences between traditional and modern foods appear to be in vitamin, mineral, and fiber content. All traditional groups ate meat regularly, which may surprise vegetarians who think theirs is the ideal diet. The meat was not what we find in our grocery stores today, however, but consisted of wild game, fish, fowl, and, occasionally, livestock. Organ meats of these animals were commonly consumed in dishes such as fish heads stuffed with liver

TABLE 2.1   DENTAL CAVITIES IN TRADITIONAL
PEOPLE, BY AVERAGE PERCENTAGE
OF TEETH AFFECTED BY CAVITIES

People	Traditional Diet	Modern Diet
Swiss	4.60%	29.8%
Gaelics	1.20	30.0
Eskimos	0.09	13.0
Northern American Indians	0.16	21.5
Seminole Indians	4.00	40.0
Melanesians	0.38	29.0
Polynesians	0.32	21.9
Africans	0.20	6.8
Australian aborigines	0.00	70.9
New Zealand Maori	0.01	55.3
Malays	0.09	20.6
Coastal Peruvians	0.04	40.0+
High Andes Indians	0.00	40.0+
Amazon Indians	0.00	40.0+

(Source: Price, 1938)

TABLE 2.2   TRADITIONAL DIETS IN WESTON PRICE'S STUDY

Traditional Alpine Swiss, isolated without roads

Diet:	Grains (mostly oats) and dairy products — milk, butter, cream, and cheese. Greens and vegetables only during the summer months. Meat from livestock once a week.
Special considerations:	The dairy cows were grass-fed, pasturing in mineral-rich wild pastures at the edge of glaciers.
Mineral source:	Glacial soil.

Isolated Gaelics, Outer Hebrides Islands

Diet:	Fish, lobster, oysters, clams, oats, barley, limited dairy products, very limited vegetables, no fruit.
Special considerations:	Organ meats from the seafood, including fish head and cod liver.
Mineral source:	The sea.

Isolated Eskimos, Northern Alaska

Diet:	Fresh and dried fish, seal oil, fish eggs, caribou, whale and seal organ meats, ground nuts, berries (preserved by freezing), flower blossoms and sorrel grass (preserved in seal oil), green sea vegetables.
Mineral source:	The sea.

North American Indians, Northern Canadian wilderness

Diet:	Wild game, limited vegetable matter in season.
Special considerations:	Extensive knowledge of the dietary and medicinal uses of the various internal organs and tissues of wild game. The muscle meat was fed to dogs.
Mineral source:	Forest-fed animals.

(continues)

TABLE 2.2 *(continued)*

North American Indians, Southern Alaska

Diet:	Seafood (including sea plants), moose and deer meat, limited vegetables, dried berries in winter.
Mineral sources:	Forest-fed animals and forest soils.

North American Indians, Florida Everglades

Diet:	Fish, wild game, wild greens, fruits, and roots.
Mineral sources:	Pristine algae-rich fresh water, forest-fed animals, and forest soils.

Isolated Melanesians, New Caledonia and the Fiji Islands

Diet:	Fish, shellfish, wild pig, wild plant foods.
Mineral sources:	The sea and forest soils.

Isolated Polynesians, Hawaiian Islands, Tahiti, and nearby islands

Diet:	Wild plant foods, supplemented by foods from the sea.
Mineral sources:	The sea and forest soils.

Masai tribe, East Africa

Diet:	Milk, blood from cattle, some meat, varying amounts of wild vegetables and fruits.
Mineral sources:	Mineral-rich blood, forest soils.

Kikuyu tribe, East Africa

Diet:	Sweet potatoes, corn, beans, millet, bananas, frogs, insects, and occasional meat from livestock.
Special considerations:	Price noted that the Kikuyu did not thrive as a tribe and were generally dominated by their neighbors.
Mineral source:	Agricultural soils prone to mineral depletion.

(continues)

TABLE 2.2 *(continued)*

Buganda tribe, East Africa

Diet:	Freshwater fish, bananas, sweet potatoes, goat's milk.
Mineral sources:	Algae-rich fresh waters, forest soils.

Australian aborigines

Diet:	Wide variety of wild foods, wild game, fish, fowl, insects, and plants. Those who lived by the sea ate a wide variety of sea animals and sea plants.
Mineral sources:	The sea, wild uncultivated soils.

New Zealand Maori

Diet:	Shellfish (especially clams), kelp, fern root, grubs, vegetables, and fruits.
Mineral sources:	The sea, wild uncultivated soils.

Ancient Peruvians (Archeological records)

Diet:	Cultivated grains, meat from livestock, sea foods.
Special considerations:	Plants fertilized with the droppings of seabirds.
Mineral source:	The sea.

Peruvian Indians

Diet:	Llama, alpaca, wild deer, birds, guinea pigs, dried fish eggs, and sea kelp (even among the high-altitude Indians).
Mineral sources:	The sea, forest-fed animals, uncultivated natural soils.

Amazon Indians

Diet:	Fish, wild game, wild birds, wild bird eggs, wild vegetables, and fruits.
Mineral sources:	Forest-fed game, forest soils.

---

among the Gaelics, selected organs of sea mammals by the Eskimos, or brains, eyes, bone marrow, and other organs by the Canadian Indians. The Canadian Indians fed the muscle meat of deer to their dogs. Several East African tribes used (and still use) blood from cattle as a major food. Blood is especially rich in minerals. Other special foods included fish and bird eggs, insects, and medicinal plants. Plant foods included wild roots, greens, fruits, berries, sea vegetables, and grains grown in mineral-rich soils. Plants containing special nutrients were also used for medicinal purposes. In Africa, for example, the water hyacinth, which is rich in iodine, was used to cure goiter.

THE MODERN FOODS

The modern foods that wreaked such havoc on the health of indigenous people were the same ones we eat regularly today: sugar, refined flour, canned food, domesticated meats, and cultivated rather than wild vegetables. In each section following, I'll describe the kind of nutrient deficiencies that inevitably follow a shift in diet from natural to processed foods. I'll also discuss these in more detail in Section 3, "Getting the Minerals You Need."

Sugar

Sugar presents a number of problems nutritionally. By itself, sugar depresses the immune system (Bernstein, 1977; Sanchez et al, 1973; Ringsdorf et al, 1976). When this happens, the body needs more immune system–supporting vitamins and minerals, such as vitamins A, B_{12}, and C, as well as folic acid, pantothenic acid, pyridoxine, riboflavin, copper, and zinc (Werbach, 1993). The most devastating effect of sugar consumption as a major calorie source is that the body is robbed of the nutrients that would accompany those calories if whole food were consumed instead. Table 2.3 shows the nutrients that are lost by taking five hundred calories from sugar rather than from the whole oats eaten by the alpine Swiss in Price's study. The loss amounts to between one-half and one-third the required daily intake of protein, half the daily healthy intake of fiber, half the required daily intake of iron, and most of the daily intake of

TABLE 2.3   NUTRIENT LOSS IN SUGAR VS.
OATS FOR CALORIC INTAKE
(PER 500 CALORIES)

Nutrient	Whole Oats	Sugar	% Change
Protein	20.83 g	0.00 g	–100.00
Fiber	13.80 g	0.00 g	–100.00
Minerals			
Calcium	67.71 mg	1.29 mg	–98.09
Iron	5.47 mg	0.08 mg	–98.58
Magnesium	192.71 mg	0.00 mg	–100.00
Phosphorus	617.19 mg	2.58 mg	–99.58
Potassium	455.73 mg	2.58 mg	–99.43
Zinc	4.00 mg	0.04 mg	–99.03
Copper	0.45 mg	0.06 mg	–87.56
Manganese	4.73 mg	0.01 mg	–99.81
Vitamins			
Thiamine	0.95 mg	0.00 mg	–100.00
Riboflavin	0.18 mg	0.02 mg	–86.53
Niacin	1.02 mg	0.00 mg	–100.00
Vitamin B$_6$	0.16 mg	0.00 mg	–100.00
Folate	41.67 mcg	0.00 mcg	–100.00
Vitamin A	131.51 IU	0.00 IU	–100.00
Vitamin E	0.60 IU	0.00 IU	–100.00

Average nutrient loss from sugar: 98.5%

(Source: U.S. Department of Agriculture, 1997)

magnesium. The body must then metabolize the calories from the sugar, which robs the bones and tissues of the mineral co-factors metabolism requires.

Refined Flour

Several of the groups Price studied ate whole grains, and members became ill when they switched to white flour. During the flour-refining process, the tough outer husk of the grain is removed, making it sweeter but robbing it of much of its nutritional value. Table 2.4 compares the nutrients in a slices of whole wheat and white bread. I've selected the values for enriched white bread, which has minerals and vitamins added, to demonstrate how little such fortification does to offset the losses during refining. The increases in the "Percent Change" column reflect nutrients added in the enriching process.

Canned Foods

Price also noted an increasing reliance on canned foods among the groups that showed declining health. Preparing and canning vegetables and other foods often dramatically reduces their nutrient content. Table 2.5 shows the nutrients lost in the canning of peas. Also relevant to the discussion of traditional peoples eating canned vegetables is the switch from nutrient-rich wild foods and seaweeds to nutritionally inferior cultivated foods. Table 2.6 compares the nutrients in wild nettle leaves, a common traditional pot herb, and cabbage. Three ounces of nettle leaf alone provides more than the minimum daily requirement of calcium and magnesium. All wild greens are not as rich in calcium, but all have higher levels of calcium, magnesium, potassium, and the trace elements than cultivated greens. See Table 26.17.

TABLE 2.4   Nutrient Loss in White vs.
Whole Wheat Bread (1 Slice)

Nutrient	Whole Wheat	Enriched White*	% Change
Protein	9.7 g	8.2 g	–15.46
Fiber	6.9 g	2.3 g	–66.67
Minerals			
Calcium	72 mg	108 mg	+50.00
Iron	3.30 mg	3.03 mg	–8.18
Magnesium	86 mg	24 mg	–72.09
Phosphorus	229 mg	94 mg	–58.95
Potassium	252 mg	119 mg	–52.78
Zinc	1.94 mg	0.62 mg	–68.04
Copper	0.284 mg	0.126 mg	–55.63
Manganese	2.320 mg	0.383 mg	–83.49
Vitamins			
Thiamine	0.351 mg	0.472 mg	+34.47
Riboflavin	0.205 mg	0.341 mg	+66.34
Niacin	3.830 mg	3.969 mg	+3.63
Vitamin B$_6$	0.179 mg	0.064 mg	–64.25
Folate	50 mcg	34 mcg	–32.00
Vitamin B$_{12}$	0.01 mcg	0.02 mcg	+100.00
Vitamin E	6.0 IU	0.19 IU	–97.25

(Source: U.S. Department of Agriculture, 1997)

*Calcium, iron, and B vitamins added

Wild Game vs. Domestic Meat

The final change common to some of the diets that Price found in transition is a switch from wild fish and game to domestic meats. Table 2.7 compares some nutrients in domesticated beef and several species of wild game and fish. Wild game is generally higher in minerals because the animals can browse the

TABLE 2.5   NUTRIENT CONTENT IN FRESH VS.
CANNED PEAS (100 GRAMS)

Nutrient	Fresh	Canned*	% Change
Fiber	5.1 g	4.1 g	–19.60
Minerals			
Calcium	25 mg	20 mg	–20.00
Iron	1.47 mg	0.95 mg	–35.37
Magnesium	33 mg	17 mg	–48.48
Phosphorus	108 mg	67 mg	–37.96
Potassium	244 mg	173 mg	–29.10
Zinc	1.24 mg	0.71 mg	–42.74
Copper	0.176 mg	0.082 mg	–53.41
Manganese	0.410 mg	0.303 mg	–26.10
Vitamins			
Vitamin C	40 mg	9.6 mg	–76.00
Thiamine	0.266 mg	0.121 mg	–54.51
Riboflavin	0.132 mg	0.078 mg	–40.91
Niacin	2.09 mg	0.732 mg	–64.98
Vitamin B$_6$	0.104 mg	0.064 mg	–38.46
Folate	0.169 mcg	0.064 mcg	–62.13
Vitamin A	65 IU	44.3 IU	–31.85
Vitamin E	0.26 IU	0.25 IU	–2.56

Average nutrient loss: 41.54%

(Source: U.S. Department of Agriculture, 1997)

*Drained solids

TABLE 2.6   SOME MINERALS IN WILD VS.
CULTIVATED GREENS (100 GRAMS)

Mineral	Nettle Leaf	Cabbage	% Change
Calcium	966.67 mg	47.00 mg	–95.13
Magnesium	286.67 mg	15.00 mg	–94.76
Iron	1.40 mg	0.59 mg	–57.85
Potassium	583.33 mg	246.00 mg	–57.82
Manganese	0.260 mg	0.159 mg	–38.84
Zinc	0.16 mg	0.18 mg	+14.89

(Sources: Pederson, 1994, and U.S. Department of Agriculture, 1997)

TABLE 2.7   NUTRIENTS IN DOMESTIC BEEF VS. WILD GAME (100 GRAMS)

Nutrient	Beef	Deer	Elk	Bison	Salmon	% Change
Fat	19.20 g	2.42 g	1.45 g	1.84 g	6.34 g	+537.34
% EFA*	3.59	15.70	14.48	7.61	7.37	−68.17
Iron	1.85 mg	3.40 mg	2.76 mg	2.60 mg	0.80 mg	−22.59
Magnesium	19 mg	23 mg	23 mg	25 mg	29 mg	−24.00
Potassium	297 mg	318 mg	312 mg	343 mg	490 mg	−18.80
Zinc	3.66 mg	2.09 mg	2.40 mg	2.80 mg	0.64 mg	+84.62
Copper	0.07 mg	0.25 mg	0.12 mg	0.09 mg	0.25 mg	−60.73
Manganese	0.01 mg	0.04 mg	0.01 mg	0.01 mg	0.02 mg	−36.84

(Source: U.S. Department of Agriculture, 1997)

* Essential fatty acids, omega-6 and omega-3

mineral-rich plants of the forest or field. Domestic animals are more prone to mineral deficiencies because their pastures gradually become depleted of minerals. Domestic animals also carry much higher body fat. The same size portion of domesticated meat provides nearly five times as much fat as game meat or fish. The composition of that fat is also important. The essential fatty acids linoleic and alpha-linolenic acid perform a number of vital functions in the body, and their percentage as a portion of total fat determines the percentage that ends up in the cell membranes of your body. With the substitution of beef for wild game, the proportion of essential fatty acids falls by almost 70 percent.

WHAT WAS LOST

The four most prominent nutrient losses with the switch from traditional to modern foods appear to be: vitamins, minerals, fiber, and essential fatty acids. I will discuss fiber and essential fatty acids in greater detail in Section 3, "Getting the Minerals You Need." The tables in this chapter show what happened to the health of the people Weston Price studied when they switched diets. Their bellies may have been full, and they may have gotten enough caloric intake to keep their bodies running, but they were starving for vital nutrients.

In Price's assessment, the increase in sugar and refined flours and the decrease in vitamins and minerals were the most important dietary changes. He found that the traditional diets had four times the minerals and ten times the fat-soluble vitamins of modern diets (see page 201). Price did not conclude, however, that fat in the modern diet was a major source of disease—in contrast to current theories—or that meat itself was a source of disease, as some modern vegetarians hold. Price suggested that the quality of fats and meats was important, and that animal fat and marine oils, rich in fat-soluble vitamins, were an important component of a healthy diet. He also concluded that the fat-soluble vitamins A and D were necessary for the absorption of minerals. Modern diet studies validate his findings. In third world countries where poor inhabitants do not consume animal products, iron-deficiency anemia is common. There is plenty of iron in the vegetable foods the people eat, but they cannot absorb it in the absence of vitamin A. The addition of vitamin A to the diets, in the form of cod liver oil, increases iron absorption and cures the anemia. Other studies of animals showed that dogs fed primarily on whole grains did not absorb the abundant calcium in the grains until cod liver oil or butter, also rich in vitamin A, is added.

MODERN STUDIES

Although Weston Price presented strong clinical data about the relationship of diet and dental cavities, the most dramatic evidence to back his theories lies in his photographs. This kind of information is hard to quantify, however, and does not satisfy the modern scientist. But in the last thirty years a large number of more formal studies of the effect of Western diets on primitive societies have been conducted that support Price's theories. Perhaps the best summary of this research appears in *Western Diseases: Their Emergence and Prevention* by Drs. H. C. Trowell and D. P. Burkitt (1981). Both men taught and practiced medicine in Uganda (for a total of 49 teaching years between them) and saw the effects of the increasing Western influences on the diet there. Both were in retirement in 1966 when the text *Diabetes, Coronary Thrombosis and the Saccharine Disease* appeared (Cleave and Campbell, 1966), which reported that the incidence of these illnesses increases when sugar is introduced into a society's diet. Trowell and Burkitt were thus inspired to come out of retirement and invite contributions from thirty-four leading researchers in the field of dietary research for a text on the subject. After preliminary research, they presented the researchers with a list of twenty-five diseases that scientific studies had suggested were Western diseases—illnesses that are common in the Western developed world and rare in traditional societies, but which appear in indigenous societies when individuals switch to a Western diet. Table 2.8 lists the diseases that Burkitt, Trowell, and the contributors concluded are Western diseases, brought on by the diet and lifestyle factors of modern society.

Trowell and Burkitt also noted that these diseases appeared in the traditional societies in the same order of emergence as they appear in the lifetimes of westerners. For instance, obesity occurs first and is followed by increased incidence of adult-onset diabetes. Cardiovascular diseases appear in the following order: hypertension, stroke, cardiac and renal complications of hypertension, angina pain, and myocardial infarction (heart attack). In Western societies, which have spent

TABLE 2.8   WESTERN DISEASES THAT ARE
             RARE OR NONEXISTENT IN
             TRADITIONAL SOCIETIES

Diseases	Associated Dietary Deficiencies
Metabolic and Cardiovascular	
Essential hypertension	Calcium, magnesium, potassium
Obesity	Copper, zinc
Diabetes (Type II)	Chromium, copper, magnesium, manganese, zinc
Cholesterol gallstones	Fiber
Stroke	Calcium, magnesium, potassium
Peripheral vascular disease	Calcium, chromium, copper, magnesium, selenium
Coronary heart disease	Calcium, chromium, copper, magnesium, selenium
Varicose veins	Copper
Deep vein thrombosis	Essential fatty acids
Pulmonary embolism	Essential fatty acids

(continues)

TABLE 2.8 *(continued)*

Diseases	Associated Dietary Deficiencies
Diseases of the Colon	
Constipation	Fiber
Appendicitis	Fiber
Diverticular disease	Fiber
Hemorrhoids	Fiber
Colon cancer and polyps	Fiber, calcium
Ulcerative colitis	Magnesium, zinc
Crohn's disease	Magnesium, zinc
Other	
Dental caries	Calcium, magnesium, zinc
Kidney stones	Magnesium
Pulmonary embolism	Essential fatty acids
Gout	Vitamin C
Thyrotoxicosis	None established by science
Pernicious anemia	Vitamin B_{12}
Breast cancer	Calcium, magnesium, copper, iodine, magnesium, selenium, and zinc
Prostate cancer	Calcium, magnesium, copper, iodine, magnesium, selenium, and zinc
Ovarian cancer	Calcium, magnesium, copper, iodine, magnesium, selenium, and zinc
Rheumatoid arthritis	Copper, selenium, sulfur, zinc
Osteoarthritis	Boron, selenium, sulfur, zinc

(Sources: Appleton, 1996; Trowell and Burkitt, 1981; Werbach, 1993)

the last ten thousand years gradually shedding traditional diets, the end stages of cardiovascular disease are among our leading causes of death.

RISK FACTORS IN THE WESTERN DIET

The risk factors for the diseases that Trowell and Burkitt name are: low fiber, high fat, sugar, and high salt in the diet. They do not discuss mineral deficiencies as causative factors, but most of these factors are related to mineral intake. Plants that are high in fiber are also high in minerals. High sugar intake provides calories without the minerals that would accompany the calories in whole foods. The body then must rob its internal tissue's mineral stores to metabolize those calories. I'll discuss the effects of sodium in Chapter 12. Trowell and Burkitt's association of high fat with Western disease contradicts Price's observation, and has also been criticized by other researchers (Fallon and Enig, 1997).

My guess is that the reason Burkitt, Trowell, and the other researchers did not discuss the changes in mineral content between primitive and Western diets is that recent discoveries in mineral nutrition had not caught up with them. Box 2.1 shows the year the essential intake of each trace mineral was the discovered. A so-called "forty-year rule" in medicine holds that new medical knowledge takes about forty years to become integrated into standard practice. True to the rule, the anticancer effects of selenium, which was proven essential to life in 1957, are being broadcast as a "breakthrough" in the media as I write this in 1997. At the time Trowell, Burkitt, and their associates were writing in the mid-seventies, the knowledge of the essentiality of the minerals lower on the list than the cobalt in vitamin B_{12} had probably not filtered into their thinking. Zinc, which was known to be essential for animals in 1934, was not recognized as an essential human nutrient until the 1970s. Besides these known essential trace minerals, others such as arsenic, fluoride, lithium, bromide, germanium, and rubidium are known to have benefits for life in small doses (Nielsen, 1996). The depletion of this whole spectrum of trace elements in the Western diet probably contributes to the emergence of Western diseases. You will learn about the individual role of the minerals in health and disease, and their connection to the most common illnesses in our society, in Section 2, "Minerals in Health and Disease."

BOX 2.1

SOME BENEFICIAL TRACE ELEMENTS BY YEAR OF RECOGNITION*

Iron	17th century	Chromium	1959
		Tin	1970
Iodine	19th century	Vanadium	1971
		Fluorine	1971
Copper	1928	Silicon	1972
Manganese	1931	Nickel	1964
Zinc	1934	Arsenic	1975
Cobalt	1935	Cadmium	1977
Molybdenum	1953	Lead	1977
Selenium	1957	Boron	1990

(Sources: Lenihan, 1988; Nielsen, 1996; Wallach and Lan, 1994)

*Benefits demonstrated in animals, but not necessarily humans

CONCLUSION

In *Nutrition and Physical Degeneration*, Weston Price included a chapter on the problem of the agricultural depletion of minerals in the soil and the food that comes from it. He even introduced preliminary data showing a correlation between regional soil-mineral depletion and the incidence of heart disease and pneumonia. In the next chapter, I'll discuss soil depletion and its impact on the mineral content in the foods we eat today. In Chapter 4, I'll show the impact mineral depletion of our foods has on our health as a nation.

CHAPTER 3

The Food Chain Broken: The Crisis in Modern Nutrition

We didn't inherit the land from our fathers. We are borrowing it from our children.

Amish belief

In Chapter 1, I described how minerals move up the food chain. In this chapter, I'll explain how modern agriculture has broken that food chain, and I'll show the impact that has had on the mineral content of your food.

AN APPLE A DAY

The saying "An apple a day keeps the doctor away" became popular in the United States in the early part of this century. But the expression goes back much further than that, and is repeated in many languages and cultures. A contemporary Arabic version is: "An apple a day will keep away a thousand doctors."

Growing up as a child in the 1940s and 1950s, I often wondered what was so special about apples. My father was a medical doctor, and I was familiar with hospitals, operations, the extent of illness in the United States, and the genuine need for doctors' expertise. It seemed unimaginable that apples could prevent illness. I didn't realize this statement's roots in truth until I began researching mineral-nutrient data for this book.

Table 3.1 shows the decline in the mineral content of apples between 1914 and 1992. Table 3.2 shows the decline in vitamin content from 1963 to 1992. Vitamin data is not available

TABLE 3.1   EIGHTY-YEAR DECLINE IN
             MINERAL CONTENT OF ONE
             MEDIUM APPLE (RAW, WITH SKIN)

Mineral	1914	1963	1992	% Change (1914–1992)
Calcium	13.5 mg	7.0 mg	7.0 mg	−48.15
Phosphorus	45.2 mg	10.0 mg	7.0 mg	−84.51
Iron	4.6 mg	0.3 mg	0.18 mg	−96.09
Potassium	117.0 mg	110.0 mg	115.0 mg	−1.71
Magnesium	28.9 mg	8.0 mg	5.0 mg	−82.70

(Source: Lindlaar, 1914; USDA, 1963 and 1997)

TABLE 3.2   CHANGES IN THE VITAMIN CONTENT
             OF ONE MEDIUM APPLE
             (RAW, WITH SKIN)

Vitamin	1963	1992	% Change
Vitamin A	90 IU	53 IU	−41.11
Vitamin C	4 mg	5.7 mg	+42.50
Thiamine	0.03 mg	0.017 mg	−43.33
Riboflavin	0.02 mg	0.014 mg	−30.00
Niacin	0.1 mg	0.077 mg	−23.00

(Source: USDA, 1963 and 1997)

from 1914, because most vitamins had not been discovered yet. Apples, as they were grown when the "apple a day" saying was coined, contained significant mineral and vitamin nutrition. An apple in the United States in 1914 contained almost half the minimum daily requirement of iron. Today's apples contain less than one-fiftieth of the requirement—you'd have to eat twenty-six apples to get the same iron nutrition from one apple today. I will describe similar nutrient losses for many foods later in this chapter (see Tables 3.7 to 3.12). Figure 3.1 shows the decline in mineral content of a group of vegetables since 1914.

SOIL MINERAL DEPLETION

So where did the all the minerals go in eighty years? They disappeared from the soil. In a stable ecosystem, minerals are drawn from the soil into the plants as they grow and bear fruit. When the plant dies, the minerals return to the earth for other plants to use. However, if the farmer hauls away the plants or their fruits and grains with a harvest, the minerals in them are removed from the cycle. The soil then becomes gradually depleted of its minerals, unless more are added to it in the form of fertilizers. Most soils will support only about ten years of intensive farming before the land becomes so mineral-depleted that it will no longer produce healthy plants.

Knowledge of soil depletion is as ancient as agriculture itself. About ten thousand years ago, hunter-gatherers began to plant food crops, perhaps in cleared areas of the forest. When the land began to fail, they would simply clear a new plot and plant there, letting nature reclaim the original land. Some primitive agricultural people still practice these methods today. They cut and burn away plots of the forest to grow their crops. The ash from the burned plants acts as a mineral fertilizer to enrich the soil until it eventually becomes barren.

METHODS THAT MAINTAIN THE SOIL

As farmers settled on permanent plots of land, they developed ways to restore the mineral content of the soil. They would use plant or manure fertilizers on the soil to restore some of the nutrients. Plant matter used for fertilizer replaces the plant matter taken away in the crops, keeping a balance in the mineral cycle of the soil. The manure of grazing animals returns some of the minerals from the forage crops where the animals graze. In some cultures, farmers ground up the mineral-rich bones of dead animals to enrich the soil. For centuries in Asia, even up to the present day, farmers have returned animal and even human waste to the soil. In some areas, such as the Nile River valley, periodic flooding covers the farmland with new mineral-rich soil from upstream. This phenomenon has made the Nile valley a source of the most highly nutritious foods in the entire Mediterranean region since ancient times. The love story of Anthony and Cleopatra takes place during the Roman conquest of the rich agricultural regions of Egypt after their own farmlands became depleted.

Crop rotation is another method for remineralizing the soil. Medieval English farm communities allowed one-third of the crop land to lie fallow each year, and all the manure from the grazing animals was put into the soil of that land. Another third lay fallow the next year, and crops were planted in the soil fertilized the year before. This system slows the mineral decline in the soil, but does not stop it completely. Pastureland also eventually becomes mineral-depleted, as the animals use the minerals and as the manure is systematically hauled away. The herd eventually thins, the forage plants become mineral-depleted, and the fallow land ultimately becomes barren as well. In Britain, the pastures were wasted, the cows became scrawny, and their droppings ceased to fertilize the gardens. This agricultural decline was one of many factors in the movement from the farm to the city in Britain over the last two hundred years.

Farmers may also plant certain non-cash crops on their fallow land and then plow the crops under. Some farmers today plant alfalfa in their fallow fields every four years. Alfalfa has deep roots that may extend more than twenty feet down into the soil. These roots bring up minerals from the deeper layers of the soil, which are returned to the topsoil when the crop is plowed under. This method also eventually fails, perhaps after centuries, when the deeper layers of the soil also become depleted of minerals.

This traditional method of crop rotation with plant and animal fertilizers today is called *organic farming*. It is traditional farming using the same methods that have sustained farm communities for many centuries to produce nutrient-rich foods.

SOIL DECLINE IN AMERICAN HISTORY

With subsistence farming, where the family or community takes only what they need for personal use from the soil, the process of depletion may take hundreds or even thousands of years. With the advent of urbanization and the demand for food crops by city dwellers, commercial rather than subsistence agriculture becomes predominant, more plants are hauled away from the soil, and the soil mineral loss accelerates. The urbanization of the United States in the last century has contributed greatly to the dramatic soil depletion indicated by the mineral data for apples in Tables 3.1 and 3.2. At the turn of the last century, about 85 percent of the population lived on farms, grew much of the food they ate, and practiced crop rotation. Today, more than 85 percent of the population lives in cities and requires food from land cared for and tended to by someone else, and to which the consumers themselves do not return their wastes. The mineral cycle of the land is broken. Instead of being returned to the land, our mineral wastes now go into landfills and sewers. Plants whose minerals were so carefully guarded and returned to the soil by subsistence farmers for millennia are now shipped overseas at a rate of more than 100 million tons per year (U.S. Department of Commerce, 1996). Table 3.3, which compares the dollar volume of U.S. food exports between 1970 and 1992, shows the rapid recent acceleration of this process.

The burned-out farm has been a part of American history since well before the first Europeans arrived here. Anthropologists think that soil depletion may have been responsible for the decline or disappearance of some corn-farming communities in the Southwest. Weston Price, the dentist who studied the effects of traditional diets introduced in Chapter 2, also found anthropological evidence of progressive soil decline in the lands of Southwestern Indians. He examined skeletons from a period of more than a thousand years and found an increase in arthritis, tooth decay, and degeneration of bone structure in progressive generations. These communities hunted but also grew corn, and Price speculates that it was the progressive depletion of minerals in the soil the corn was grown in that caused the gradual decline in health.

Soil depletion also fueled the historic westward expansion of the United States. As the colonists' land became depleted,

TABLE 3.3   ANNUAL EXPORT OF FOOD CROPS
FROM THE UNITED STATES

Year	Amount
1970	$7,255,000,000
1980	$41,200,000,000
1992	$45,700,000,000

(Source: U.S. Department of Commerce, 1989 and 1994)

they abandoned it to look for new land to the west. This phenomenon also influenced the movement from rural areas to cities. A few cultures—those that used wise agricultural methods—did not have to leave their land. In areas of Pennsylvania, Germans, the Amish, and other groups still farm land today that their ancestors settled more than a hundred years ago. These groups believe that the soil they leave their children should be healthier than the soil they inherited. Some German settlers even took over burned-out farms and restored the soil to health (Ebeling, 1979).

Weston Price noted the general decline of minerals in the soil by 1938:

In correspondence with government officials in practically every state of the United States I find that during the last fifty years there has been a reduction in the capacity of the soil for productivity in many districts, amounting from 25 to 50 percent. (Price, 1938)

Price also found a correspondence between soil depletion in specific areas and an increased incidence of heart disease and pneumonia in those areas.

THE RISE OF NPK FERTILIZER

Soil depletion continues to play an important role in the unfolding history of the family farm in the United States. Traditional farming methods have been abandoned in favor of intensive use of chemical fertilizers in the last thirty years. NPK fertilizer— named from the chemical symbols for nitrogen, phosphorus, and potassium—has largely replaced manures, organic plant material, and ground up animal bones as fertilizer on commercial farms. Table 3.4 shows the nutrients required by plants. Of these, the primary nutrients nitrogen, phosphorus, and potassium are most responsible for the growth, size, and productivity of agricultural crops, and thus they are the primary elements of modern fertilizers like NPK.

The deficiency of a few nutrients—sulfur and iron, for example—will cause discoloration of plants, affecting their marketability (Stewart, 1977). The other elements are less crucial to productivity or appearance, although they are extremely important to the nutritional value of the plants to humans. If the secondary nutrients or trace elements become so depleted that it affects the productivity or appearance of a crop, these nutrients may be added to the soil. For instance, iron is often added to fertilizers for commercial potato crops, which rapidly deplete the soil of the iron essential to the growth and appearance of the potato. The U.S. Department of Agriculture assists farmers in determining whether additional nutrients need to be added to soil to support plant growth, productivity, and appearance. The nutritional value of the food is not considered in such analyses. Plants remove all these nutrients from the soil, but contemporary farmers add only three or four minerals back in. If you look ahead to Table 3.13, you'll see how, of the five minerals listed, phosphorus and potassium have declined the least in foods since 1963. This is because these two minerals are standard ingredients in modern fertilizers. NPK fertilizer was developed in the 1830s before we understood the mineral requirements of either plants or humans. We are using an outdated technology, despite what modern scientific knowledge has taught us about the nutritional value of minerals.

The effect of chemical fertilizers is more complex than simple mineral loss. The addition of chemical nitrogen depletes both the vitamin C and the iron content of plants that grow

TABLE 3.4   PLANT NUTRIENT REQUIREMENTS

Nutrients	Source
Organic elements	*Air and water*
hydrogen	
oxygen	
carbon	
Primary nutrients	*Soil*
nitrogen	
phosphorus	
potassium	
Secondary nutrients	*Soil*
magnesium	
calcium	
sulfur	
Trace elements	*Soil*
iron	
zinc	
manganese	
boron	
copper	
molybdenum	
chlorine	

(Source: Donahue, 1970)

from the fertilized soil (Harris, 1975). In addition, the potassium in NPK fertilizer is added in the form of potassium chloride, which means a ton of chloride is added along with every ton of potassium. The high levels of potassium inhibit plant absorption of magnesium (Ensminger et al., 1983). Chloride leaches the soil of magnesium, zinc, and calcium (Hall, 1976).

Potassium chloride also alters the mineral balance so that selenium becomes bound in the soil and cannot be absorbed by plants (Ensminger et al., 1983).

PESTICIDES AND FUNGICIDES

The result of decades of farming with NPK fertilizer is that plants look the same as they did generations ago, but they are depleted of the secondary plant nutrients and trace elements. Although the yield is adequate for commercial purposes, these plants are diseased. Plants, like humans, can suffer from mineral-deficiency symptoms that affect their immune systems (Salamon, 1974; Fryer, 1984). They are more prone to mold, fungus, and insect infestation, and they require large quantities of pesticides to keep them alive until they reach the market. So besides being inferior in mineral content, modern agricultural products are laced with potentially poisonous substances. Table 3.5 shows the increasing farm expenditures for fertilizer and pesticides since 1970. During this period, the average units of fertilizer and pesticides per acre of harvested cropland have increased about 25 percent (U.S. Department of Commerce, 1989 and 1996).

TABLE 3.5   EXPENDITURES FOR FERTILIZER
AND PESTICIDES ON U.S.
FARMS, 1970–1994
(IN BILLIONS OF DOLLARS)

Year	Fertilizer	Pesticides
1970	2.4	1.0
1987	6.5	4.6
1994	9.2	7.2

(Source: U.S. Department of Commerce, 1989 and 1996)

THE ECOLOGY OF SOIL MICROORGANISMS

We learned in Chapter 1 that soil microorganisms are a key link in the mineralization of soil. They may ingest minerals from rocks in the soil, and they break down the organic matter of dead plants, rereleasing their minerals for use by other plants. Table 3.6 shows the forms of microscopic life in soil that are essential to mineral transformation and retention in soil. Each teaspoon of healthy soil contains a complex microscopic ecology; the presence of each of the life forms is necessary for the maintenance of soil fertility and mineral transformation. Minerals ingested by fungi and bacteria may not be available to plants, but the tiny predatory protozoa, nematodes, and microarthropods eat bacteria, fungi, and each other, and release their nutrients in fecal matter (Ingham, 1985, 1992).

Chemical fertilizers and pesticides kill many of these beneficial organisms by providing an unbalanced nutrient supply. The fertilizers can produce large plant yields for a while, but they eventually ruin the soil by disrupting the balance of the microorganisms—effectively killing them off. The bacteria and fungi hold the soil together, so once they're greatly depleted or gone soil erosion carries more nutrients away into surface or ground water (Hendrix et al., 1986; Coleman et al., 1992).

TABLE 3.6   BENEFICIAL ORGANISMS PRESENT
            IN 1 TEASPOON OF HEALTHY SOIL

Organism	Number Present
bacteria	360,000+
fungi	60,000
protozoa	100,000
nematodes	500
microarthropods	200,000

(Source: Ingham, 1985, 1992)

Pesticides affect the soil much the same way that overuse of antibiotics affects humans. At first these drugs seemed like cure-alls that could control many infectious diseases. It soon became apparent, however, that they also created resistant forms of bacteria and disrupted the healthy bacteria in the human gut. Similarly, pesticides destroy the beneficial organisms in the soil, making way for destructive organisms (such as molds) that cause disease in the plants.

EARLY HARVESTING AND NUTRIENT CONTENT

Modern agriculture has also developed plant strains and harvesting techniques that allow foods to be harvested before they are ripe. Perhaps the most notorious is the Red Rock tomato, developed through genetic research with federal funds in California universities. The Red Rock tomato is especially hard, allowing it to be harvested with machines. It then ripens on the way to market and while in storage. This tomato, and the many other plants that now ripen after, instead of before, harvesting, no longer have roots in the ground as they ripen. Mineral content in plants such as snap beans, grapes, and many greens rises during ripening if the plant has access to the minerals in the soil. Vitamin content also rises in many plants as they near ripeness (Lee and Chichester, 1974). These nutrients are deficient in the foods that are harvested before they ripen.

THE SMOKING GUN: MINERAL DEPLETION IN OUR FOODS

These facts about the effects of modern commercial agriculture on the nutrient content of plants have been known for decades. Actual measurements of the changes in nutrient content of foods over time are much harder to find, however. Searching the computer archive of the National Library of Medicine in

Bethesda, Maryland, dating back to 1966, I was unable to find a single article tracking such changes. Other references described the problem in general, but none contained comparative data. Tables 3.7 through 3.12 give some comparisons for major categories of farm products. The data in the charts compares U.S. Department of Agriculture data from an out-of-print 1963 book with USDA information now available on the Internet. The tables list the content of five minerals, plus, in some cases, vitamin content. In 1963, only five minerals—calcium, iron, magnesium, phosphorus, and potassium—were measured. Iron was the only trace element measured then, although current analyses also measure zinc, molybdenum, and copper. The USDA does not measure food levels of the other fifteen essential trace elements, but we will assume that they follow the same pattern of decline as the other minerals because they are not generally added to commercial fertilizers.

Fruits

Table 3.7 shows the changes in the nutritional value of some fruits. All the nutrients except potassium and vitamin C have declined consistently. Potassium is added to fertilizers. The inconsistent changes in vitamin C may be due to variations in the samples used. The vitamin content of fruits and vegetables varies widely within a season depending on when they are picked. Vitamins are also less susceptible to loss than minerals because the plant can make its own vitamins but must take minerals from the soil. Despite this, the vitamin A content in the three fruits declined by 66 percent. That means you'd have to eat three pieces of these fruits to get the same amount of vitamin A you got from one piece in 1963. Of the minerals, the trace element iron took the biggest hit, with a 57 percent decline. This is an ominous sign, because the other eighteen essential trace elements may have followed the same pattern.

TABLE 3.7   CHANGES IN MINERAL AND
VITAMIN CONTENT OF FRUITS,
1963–1992 (PER 100 GRAMS)

	1963	1992	% Change
Oranges			
calcium	41 mg	40 mg	–2.44
iron	0.4 mg	0.1 mg	–75.00
magnesium	11 mg	10 mg	–9.09
phosphorus	20 mg	14 mg	–30.00
potassium	200 mg	181 mg	–9.50
vitamin A	200 IU	21 IU	–89.50
vitamin C	50 mg	53 mg	+6.00
Apples			
calcium	7 mg	7 mg	0.00
iron	0.3 mg	0.18 mg	–40.00
magnesium	8 mg	5 mg	–37.50
phosphorus	10 mg	7 mg	–30.00
potassium	110 mg	115 mg	+4.55
vitamin A	90 IU	53 IU	–41.11
vitamin C	4 mg	5.7 mg	–42.50
Bananas			
calcium	8 mg	6 mg	–25.00
iron	0.7 mg	0.31 mg	–55.71
magnesium	33 mg	29 mg	–12.12
phosphorus	26 mg	20 mg	–23.08
potassium	370 mg	396 mg	+7.03
vitamin A	190 IU	81 IU	–57.37
vitamin C	10 mg	9.1 mg	–9.00

(Source: USDA, 1963 and 1997)

Vegetables

The mineral content of vegetables also declined, on the average, for all the elements that are not added to fertilizers (see

TABLE 3.8   CHANGES IN THE MINERAL
CONTENT OF VEGETABLES,
1963–1992 (PER 100 GRAMS)

	1963	1992	% Change
Carrot, raw, with skin			
calcium	37 mg	27 mg	–27.03
iron	0.7 mg	0.5 mg	–28.57
magnesium	23 mg	15 mg	–34.78
phosphorus	36 mg	44 mg	+22.22
potassium	341 mg	323 mg	–5.28
Potatoes, raw, whole			
calcium	7 mg	7 mg	0.00
iron	0.6 mg	0.76 mg	+26.67
magnesium	34 mg	21 mg	–38.24
phosphorus	53 mg	46 mg	–13.21
potassium	407 mg	543 mg	+33.42
Corn, sweet yellow, raw			
calcium	3 mg	2 mg	–33.33
iron	0.7 mg	0.52 mg	–25.71
magnesium	48 mg	37 mg	–22.92
phosphorus	111 mg	89 mg	–19.82
potassium	280 mg	270 mg	–3.57
Tomatoes			
calcium	13 mg	5 mg	–33.33
iron	0.50 mg	0.45 mg	–25.71
magnesium	14 mg	11 mg	–22.92
phosphorus	27 mg	24 mg	–19.82
potassium	244 mg	222 mg	–3.57
Celery			
calcium	39 mg	40 mg	+2.56
iron	0.3 mg	0.4 mg	+33.33
magnesium	22 mg	11 mg	–50.00
phosphorus	28 mg	25 mg	–10.71
potassium	341 mg	287 mg	–15.84

(Source: USDA, 1963 and 1997)

Table 3.8). The only dramatic increases were the phosphorus in apples, the potassium in potatoes, and the iron in potatoes and celery. Phosphorus and potassium are added to all fertilizers, and iron is added to fertilizer for certain soils and crops. Magnesium content declined the most with a 35 percent loss.

Leafy Green Vegetables

Leafy green vegetables are promoted in virtually every nutrition book as a good source of calcium, but they may not be anymore. The calcium content of the five greens in Table 3.9 has dropped by 46.4 percent in the last generation. If we exclude iceberg lettuce—which is not a very good source of calcium anyway—the average drop is 57 percent. Collard greens, originally the highest source on the list, have lost more than 85 percent of their calcium. Again excluding iceberg lettuce, the iron content of all the greens has dropped an average of 41.5 percent, perhaps indicating a similar decline in the other essential trace elements.

Beans

The mineral content of beans did not decline as severely as that of the fruits and vegetables, perhaps because the bean stalks are plowed back into the earth, reducing the mineral loss in the soil (see Table 3.10). Nevertheless, all the minerals in beans declined except the potassium and phosphorus, which is added in fertilizers.

Grains

The mineral content of grains declined less consistently than that in fruit, vegetables, and beans. Wheat, the most intensively farmed of the grains, saw a loss of all the minerals, even

TABLE 3.9   CHANGES IN MINERAL CONTENT
IN LEAFY GREEN VEGETABLES,
1963–1992 (PER 100 GRAMS)

	1963	1992	% Change
Broccoli, raw			
calcium	103 mg	48 mg	–53.40
iron	1.10 mg	0.88 mg	–20.00
magnesium	24 mg	25 mg	+4.17
phosphorus	78 mg	66 mg	–15.38
potassium	382 mg	325 mg	–14.92
Romaine lettuce			
calcium	68 mg	36 mg	–47.06
iron	1.4 mg	1.1 mg	–21.43
magnesium	n/a*	6 mg	n/a
phosphorus	25 mg	45 mg	+80.00
potassium	264 mg	290 mg	+9.85
Iceberg lettuce			
calcium	20 mg	19 mg	–5.00
iron	0.5 mg	0.5 mg	0.00
magnesium	11 mg	9 mg	–18.18
phosphorus	22 mg	20 mg	–9.09
potassium	175 mg	158 mg	–9.71
Collard greens			
calcium	203 mg	29 mg	–85.71
iron	1.00 mg	0.19 mg	–81.00
magnesium	57 mg	9 mg	–84.21
phosphorus	63 mg	10 mg	–84.13
potassium	401 mg	169 mg	–57.86
Swiss chard			
calcium	88 mg	51 mg	–42.05
iron	3.2 mg	1.8 mg	–43.75
magnesium	65 mg	81 mg	+24.62
phosphorus	39 mg	46 mg	+17.95
potassium	550 mg	379 mg	–31.09

(Source: USDA, 1963 and 1997)

*Information not available

TABLE 3.10   CHANGES IN THE MINERAL
CONTENT OF BEANS, 1963–1992
(PER 100 GRAMS)

	1963	1992	% Change
Pintos			
calcium	135 mg	121 mg	–10.37
iron	6.4 mg	5.88 mg	–8.13
magnesium	170 mg	159 mg	–6.47
phosphorus	457 mg	418 mg	–8.53
potassium	984 mg	1,328 mg	+34.96
Chickpeas (garbanzos)			
calcium	150 mg	105 mg	–30.00
iron	6.9 mg	6.24 mg	–9.57
magnesium	n/a*	115	n/a
phosphorus	331 mg	366 mg	+10.57
potassium	797 mg	875 mg	+9.79

(Source: USDA, 1963 and 1997)

*Information not available

those that are supplied in fertilizers. In the grains listed in Table 3.11, calcium declined the most, with a loss of 46.5 percent. Grains are less susceptible to mineral loss than some other crops because the stubble of the grain is plowed back into the earth.

Meats

The mineral decline in beef and chicken, the two most frequently consumed meats in the United States, was not as dramatic as that in plants (see Table 3.12). There has been some decline, however, because the animals are fed increasingly mineral-deficient grains. But animals, like people, require minimum quantities of minerals to stay alive, so we would expect more constant levels. The most striking nutrient decline is that

TABLE 3.11   CHANGES IN THE MINERAL
              CONTENT OF GRAINS, 1963–1992
              (PER 100 GRAMS)

	1963	1992	% Change
Wheat, red winter, hard			
calcium	46 mg	29 mg	–36.96
phosphorus	354 mg	288 mg	–18.64
iron	3.40 mg	3.19 mg	–6.18
potassium	370 mg	363 mg	–1.89
magnesium	160 mg	126 mg	–21.25
Oats, rolled			
calcium	53 mg	52 mg	–1.89
phosphorus	405 mg	474 mg	+17.04
iron	4.5 mg	4.2 mg	–6.67
potassium	352 mg	350 mg	–0.57
magnesium	169 mg	148 mg	–12.43
Buckwheat			
calcium	114 mg	18 mg	–84.21
phosphorus	282 mg	347 mg	+23.05
iron	3.1 mg	2.2 mg	–29.03
potassium	448 mg	460 mg	+2.68
magnesium	229 mg	231 mg	+0.87
White rice			
calcium	24 mg	9 mg	–62.50
phosphorus	94 mg	108 mg	+14.89
iron	0.8 mg	0.8 mg	0.00
potassium	92 mg	86 mg	–6.52
magnesium	28 mg	35 mg	+25.00

(Source: USDA, 1963 and 1997)

of vitamin A, which disappeared completely from beef and declined by 70 percent in chicken, according to USDA tests. Thiamine, one of the B vitamins, declined by an average of 42 percent. Of the minerals, iron declined the most at an average

TABLE 3.12   CHANGES IN NUTRIENT CONTENT
OF BEEF AND CHICKEN,
1963–1992 (PER 100 GRAMS)

	1963	1992	% Change
Beef, ground			
calcium	10 mg	8 mg	–20.00
iron	2.70 mg	1.73 mg	–35.93
magnesium	17 mg	16 mg	–5.88
phosphorus	156 mg	130 mg	–16.67
potassium	236 mg	228 mg	–3.39
vitamin A	40 IU	0	–100.00
thiamine	0.080 mg	0.038 mg	–52.50
riboflavin	0.160 mg	0.151 mg	–5.63
niacin	4.30 mg	4.48 mg	+4.19
Chicken			
calcium	12 mg	10 mg	–16.67
phosphorus	203 mg	198 mg	–2.46
iron	1.30 mg	1.03 mg	–20.77
potassium	285 mg	238 mg	–16.49
magnesium	23 mg	23 mg	0.00
vitamin A	150 IU	45 IU	–70.00
thiamine	0.100 mg	0.069 mg	–31.00
riboflavin	0.120 mg	0.134 mg	+11.67
niacin	7.70 mg	7.87 mg	+2.21

(Source: USDA, 1963 and 1997)

of 28 percent. This may predict a similar decline in the other trace elements that the USDA does not measure. Beef has been recommended as an iron tonic for several centuries, but that advice seems to ring hollow now.

The Averages

Despite the general decline in minerals and vitamins over the years, some nutrient levels actually rose in some of the foods. The increases could be due to anything from minerals in the fertilizers, supplements given to animals, or natural variations in the sampling of the products tested. Foods grown in different soils tend to have different mineral content. Overall, though, Tables 3.7 through 3.12 show a net loss in minerals and some vitamins. Table 3.13 shows the average mineral loss for a group of fruits and vegetables. Phosphorus and potassium declined the least, because they are added to fertilizers. Iron declined the most—an ominous sign for other unmeasured essential trace elements that may have followed the same pattern. Calcium and magnesium also declined significantly. This may be due to a combination of mineral loss in the soil and chemical interactions with potassium chloride, a basic constituent of modern chemical fertilizers. Potassium inhibits plant absorption of magnesium, and chloride combines with both calcium and magnesium, leaching them from the soil.

USDA FOOD COMPOSITION DATA

In the tables in this chapter, I have given the dates for some of the data as 1963 and 1992. The current USDA information may

TABLE 3.13   CHANGES IN THE MINERAL
             CONTENT OF SOME FRUITS AND
             VEGETABLES, 1963–1992*

Mineral	Average % Change
Calcium	–29.82
Iron	–32.00
Magnesium	–21.08
Phosphorous	–11.09
Potassium	–6.48

*Fruits and vegetables measured: oranges, apples, bananas, carrots, potatoes, corn, tomatoes, celery, romaine lettuce, broccoli, iceberg lettuce, collard greens, and chard

actually include some 1963 data, and other data from the years 1976 through 1992. The bible of nutritionists and dieticians since 1963 has been the USDA's *Food Handbook No. 8*. Although the book was reprinted in 1975, it simply reproduced the 1963 data published twelve years before. Most popular nutrition books today, and even academic nutrition texts from the late 1980s, contain this thirty-four-year-old information. Shortly after the publication of the 1975 handbook, the USDA began publishing supplements as new food analyses were performed, usually on one food group at a time. Twenty-four supplements to the handbook have been printed. These supplements are now all out of print and unavailable. According to the manager of the government printing office in Denver, Colorado, no plans have been made to reprint them. The only remaining source of the data is the USDA's nutrient database—known as *SR11*—available on the Internet. It took me weeks of wrestling with bureaucracies and computer software to obtain the current information. The sources for *SR11* include some of the 1963 data and other data from various analyses performed between 1976 and 1992. So the bad news is that the 1992 entries in this chapter—dated according to the most recent USDA publication—may actually contain much older data. The food you buy in the store may have nutrient content even lower than the most recent figures in my tables. The data on fruit may come from 1982, vegetables from 1984, beans from 1986, and so on.

TRACE ELEMENTS

As I have mentioned in the discussions of the food groups, the USDA did not collect information on any of the trace elements except iron in 1963. But we have evidence that twenty-three trace elements may be beneficial to human life. Of these, the 1997 USDA nutrition database contains information on only copper, iron, molybdenum, and zinc. I was able to find analytical data on some trace elements in food from 1948. Rutgers University professor Firman E. Bear performed the research, and his data was reprinted in the 1982 book *The Survival of Civilization* by John Hamaker. Bear did not take a wide sampling of foods and publish their averages, as the USDA does. Instead, he published the high and low figures from his own and from other published analyses, showing the wide range of these elements that appear in food depending on the soil in which they are grown. Table 3.14 shows Bear's data and compares it to the 1997 USDA data. For all three trace elements listed for all five foods, the 1997 levels (from analyses in 1992 or before) are *all near or below the lowest measured in 1948.*

The implications of these data are enormous. First, here is solid evidence that modern chemical agricultural methods are effectively strip-mining essential nutrients from the soil and from the food that is grown in it. But perhaps more important, if the pattern holds true for the other twenty trace elements recognized to be beneficial to human life, then eating these food products is leading our entire nation down the road to malnutrition and disease.

COMPARATIVE DATA FROM 1914

The only source I could find for the nutrient composition of foods prior to 1948 comes from the writings of Dr. Henry Lindlahr in 1914. Lindlahr was an osteopath and naturopath who practiced in Chicago in the first decades of the twentieth century. He ran a two hundred–bed hospital where he treated the full range of human illnesses, including mental illness, using only osteopathic manipulation, homeopathy, exercise, and diet. Lindlahr was convinced of the absolute importance of a healthy, whole-foods diet in curing chronic illnesses, and avidly read the scientific literature of his day on nutrition. He pub-

TABLE 3.14   THE WORST OF THE CROP:
DISAPPEARING TRACE ELEMENTS
IN FOOD, 1948–1992
(PER 100 GRAMS OF FOOD)

	1948 (highest)	1948 (lowest)	1992 (average)
Snap Beans			
iron	22.7 mg	1.0 mg	1.04 mg
manganese	6.0 mg	0.2 mg	0.214 mg
copper	6.9 mg	0.3 mg	0.069 mg
Cabbage			
iron	9.4 mg	2.0 mg	0.59 mg
manganese	6.0 mg	0.2 mg	0.159 mg
copper	4.80 mg	0.04 mg	0.023 mg
Lettuce			
iron	51.6 mg	0.9 mg	0.5 mg
manganese	1.3 mg	0.2 mg	0.151 mg
copper	6.0 mg	0.3 mg	0.028 mg
Tomatoes			
iron	193.8 mg	0.1 mg	0.45 mg
manganese	9.4 mg	2.0 mg	0.105 mg
copper	5.3 mg	0	0.074 mg
Spinach			
iron	158.4 mg	1.9 mg	2.71 mg
manganese	51.6 mg	0.9 mg	0.097 mg
copper	3.2 mg	0.5 mg	0.13 mg

lished a four-volume work on natural therapeutics, the third of
which is on dietetics and includes his nutrient data (Lindlahr,
1914). Lindlahr does not cite a source for the data; I assume
that he, being a very wealthy man, paid to have it done. For

each of forty-five foods, he gives the content of fats and carbo-hydrates, as well as the mineral content for calcium, chlorine, iron, magnesium, phosphorus, potassium, silicon, sodium, and sulfur. I am astounded that Lindlahr would go to such lengths to analyze these nutrients in an era when only a few vitamins and two minerals were known to be essential nutrients.

Naturally we should question the validity of data this old, but also keep in mind that basic methods for quantifying mineral elements in a substance were well known at the time. The process, still in widespread use today, had been known in the mid-1800s. I learned it in college in an advanced chemistry class in 1967. The substance is burned to ash and its mineral content is analyzed using a variety of simple chemical reactions.

Lindlahr's data remain questionable, however, because either he or his chemist apparently made a mathematical error in the chart, and his mineral data all appear to be off by a factor of ten. Adjusting for this error, most of the data on minerals fall within or just above the ranges measured by Bear forty years later (see Table 3.15; Hamaker, 1982). Measurements that are higher than Bear's ranges are nevertheless consistent with the known mineral declines from 1948 to 1992. Only Lindlahr's calcium data appear widely different from Bear's. This could be consistent with soil calcium decline due to NPK fertilizer, however, which strips calcium from the soil. NPK fertilizer was introduced in the United States in the first decades of this century, and its use has been growing steadily ever since.

Table 3.15 and Figure 3.1 show the trend of mineral decline in several foods. The shape of the curve is a descending parabola, approaching a flat line. We could question whether inaccurately high calcium data from 1914 skew the curve, but the same shaped curve emerges for the sums of any two of the minerals in the chart, even omitting calcium. The 1948, 1963, and 1992 data give the same shape, excluding the 1914 data

TABLE 3.15   DECLINE OF MINERAL CONTENT
IN SOME VEGETABLES, 1914–1992
(PER 100 GRAMS)

	1914	1948 (average)	1992
Cabbage			
Calcium	248 mg	38.75 mg	47 mg
Magnesium	66 mg	29.6 mg	15 mg
Iron	1.5 mg	5.7 mg	0.59 mg
Lettuce			
Calcium	265.5 mg	38.5 mg	19 mg
Magnesium	112 mg	31.2 mg	9 mg
Iron	94 mg	26.25 mg	0.5 mg
Spinach			
Calcium	227.3 mg	71.75 mg	99 mg
Magnesium	122 mg	125.4 mg	79 mg
Iron	64 mg	80.15 mg	2.7 mg

completely. A similar curve describes the productivity of any resource extraction industry, such as coal mining or oil drilling. Productivity begins at a high level as the first resources are extracted, drops rapidly, and then levels off as the resources become exhausted. Miners and drillers do not put resources back to replace what they take out, the way traditional subsistence farmers have for thousands of years. Modern agriculture, like a mining industry, does not replace most of the minerals it extracts, but in fact exports many of them overseas. This mineral extraction industry is gradually exhausting the land.

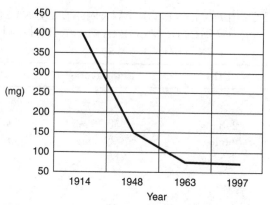

Figure 3.1   Average mineral content in selected vegetables, 1914–1997. Sums of averages of calcium, magnesium, and iron in cabbage, lettuce, tomatoes, and spinach. (Sources: Lindlahr, 1914; Hamaker, 1982; and U.S. Department of Agriculture, 1963 and 1997)

ORGANIC VEGETABLES

The growing popular appeal of organic foods is mostly due to the absence of pesticides in the plants. Whether organically grown fruits, vegetables, and grains are more nutritious than chemically grown food has been a topic of scientific debate (for a recent review of the scientific literature on the topic, see Hornick, 1992). In general, agricultural studies show little difference, on the average, between the mineral content of organically and commercially grown foods. The analyses are flawed, however, for two reasons. First, they usually compare only major minerals, excluding the trace elements. Since major minerals are often added with chemical fertilizers, the amounts in commercial produce may be equal to or higher than those in organic crops. Second, averages from across the country do not give an accurate picture. In mineral-poor farming areas, the commercial crops will have a higher concentration of the major minerals because of added fertilizers. In mineral-rich soils, with mineral-rich organic fertilizer at hand, the levels in organic crops may be higher. If the data is combined, the two trends cancel each other out, and the two types of food appear to be equal in nutritional value.

Bob L. Smith of Doctor's Data Lab in Chicago took another approach to the question in the early 1990s (Smith, 1993). For several years, he purchased organic and conventional foods in supermarkets, carefully pairing up foods of the same variety and size at the same time of year. He then had them analyzed for the content of twenty-six minerals, including twenty trace elements. Table 3.16 shows the results. On average, the organic foods have about twice the mineral content of the chemically fertilized ones. It's possible, though, that this data might not hold up if samples were taken in other areas of the country. Chicago probably gets much of its organically grown foods from farms within Illinois and neighboring states, where the crops grow in soils that are mineral-rich from glaciers that once covered the area. Of all the foods, organic corn appears to be the most rich in minerals.

CONCLUSION

The information in this chapter documents the declining mineral content of our foods that has resulted from modern agricultural methods. Our diet today—even a healthy one with plenty of fruits and vegetables—can no longer supply the minerals and vitamins that were available to our grandparents. Several minerals have declined by 20 to 30 percent in the last thirty years. To understand the impact this has on our health, consider how you would feel if you cut your calories by 20 to 30 percent, or

TABLE 3.16   NUTRIENTS IN ORGANIC VS.
COMMERCIAL FOODS*

Mineral	Organic higher	Commercial higher
boron	70%	
calcium	63	
chromium	78	
cobalt	0	
copper	48	
iodine	73	
iron		59%
lithium	116	
magnesium	136	
manganese	178	
molybdenum	68	
nickel	66	
phosphorus	91	
potassium	125	
rubidium		28
selenium	390	
silicon	86	
sodium	159	
strontium	133	
sulfur	20	
vanadium	80	
zinc		60
*Toxic trace elements** *		
aluminum		40
cadmium	5	
lead		29
mercury		25

*Nutrients higher in either organically or commercially grown apples, pears, potatoes, wheat, and corn

**With these minerals, less is better

your protein, or other key nutrients. A similar drop in key mineral nutrients is certain to have an adverse effect on your health. Perhaps the most dramatic information, contained in Table 3.15, shows the tremendous decline in trace elements, which are absolutely essential to maintain health. In the next chapter, I'll show recent trends in the incidence of diseases linked to mineral nutrition and explain why modern medicine is doing little to address the causes of these illnesses.

CHAPTER 4

TROUBLE AT THE TOP OF THE FOOD CHAIN: MINERAL DEFICIENCY DISEASES

In the last chapter, I described how modern agricultural methods demineralize the soil, putting mineral-deficient foods on your dinner table. Crops are depressed, fatigued, with depleted immune systems, overly vulnerable, and kept alive with artificial food (chemical fertilizers) and drugs (pesticides). And so are we. In this chapter, I'll show the impact this has had on the health of the nation and reveal the reasons modern medicine is not prepared to address the resulting health crisis.

THE SURGEON GENERAL'S BLIND SPOT

In 1988, U.S. Surgeon General C. Everett Koop issued a historic report on nutrition and health, the first major document by the modern medical establishment acknowledging the impact of nutrition on disease (Koop, 1988). The report described a historic change in the health of Americans in the last quarter century. According to Koop and his advisers, "Our major health problems are no longer infectious diseases or diseases associated with malnutrition, but are now those associated with dietary excesses and imbalances." The report was based on the emerging medical paradigm of "Western diseases" described in the work of Trowell and Burkitt that I introduced in Chapter 2. The "excesses and imbalances" Koop describes are excess fat, salt, and refined carbohydrates, as well as low fiber intake. The diseases of "malnutrition" he says we have outgrown are illnesses such as scurvy, caused by a gross vitamin C deficiency, or goiter, caused by too little iodine. Although Koop recommends supplementation with calcium, his report mostly overlooks the importance of minerals and trace elements, omitting information already documented by scientific literature about how the nation is suffering from a plague of mineral malnutrition. True to medicine's "forty-year rule" (see Chapter 2), Koop's report ushered U.S. health care policy from the scientific understanding of the 1930s, when gross malnutrition diseases were being recognized by science, to that of the 1940s, the decade after Weston Price so dramatically demonstrated the relationship of the Western diet to Western diseases. Koop ignored the importance of at least fifteen essential mineral and trace elements (see Table 2.9). Thus, in the years since, U.S. health care policy has been directed at reducing fat and increasing fiber in the diet, and has missed the boat on the importance of minerals.

THE MINERAL STATUS OF AMERICANS

Although the U.S. Department of Agriculture has not specifically publicized the nutrient loss in American farm products, its public reports may take those losses into account. The USDA regularly surveys Americans to determine the nutrient composition in the diets of different segments of the population. Researchers then analyze those diets for nutritional content, using the most current USDA data. Research articles based on these surveys began appearing in scientific literature of the 1980s. I have summarized some of the results following.

Calcium

- An observational study based on a 1977–1978 food-consumption survey by the USDA found that the majority of the U.S. population did not consume the recommended daily allowance (RDA) of calcium. Adult women, on average, were the most calcium-deficient group (Morgan et al., 1985).
- A review of calcium intake by the National Institutes of Health in 1984 showed that the typical American diet supplies about 450 to 550 milligrams daily, about half the RDA (NIH, 1984).
- The average American diet contains 40 to 50 percent of the RDA of calcium (Pizzorno, 1996).

Chromium

- Deficiency is common in Western diets (Anderson and Kozlovsky, 1985; Kumpulainen, 1979; Schroeder, 1968).
- Ninety percent of diets lack sufficient chromium intake (Pizzorno, 1996).

Copper

- The typical Western diet supplies only 1.0 to 1.5 milligrams of copper, significantly less than the 1.5 to 3.0

milligrams recommended daily (Schoenemann et
al., 1990).

- Seventy-five percent of American diets are copper-
deficient. The average diet contains 50 percent of the
RDA (Pizzorno, 1996).

Iron

- Iron is the most common nutrient deficient in American
children, and is frequently deficient in adolescents
(Worthington-Roberts, 1981; Armstrong, 1989).

Magnesium

- The typical American diet provides only one-half to
two-thirds of the 400 milligrams recommended daily
for magnesium; see Chapter 16 (Seelig, 1980).
- A survey of twenty-seven thousand Americans showed
that only 25 percent had a dietary intake of magnesium
that exceeded the RDA (Webster, 1987).
- Magnesium intake based on the USDA's 1977–1978
National Food Consumption Survey fell below the
RDA for all ages and both sexes, except children under
five years old (Morgan et al., 1985).
- Pregnant women often have inadequate dietary intake
of magnesium (Franz, 1987).
- Seventy-five to 85 percent of diets are magnesium-
deficient. The average diet contains 50 to 60 percent of
the RDA (Pizzorno, 1996).

Potassium

- Potassium intake is often deficient in the elderly (Abdulla et al., 1975; Touitou et al., 1987).

- Deficiency is common among hospitalized patients (Surawicz et al., 1957).

Selenium

- Selenium intake is often inadequate in Western diets (Tolonen, 1989).
- The typical selenium consumption in the United States is about 100 micrograms per day. Two to three hundred micrograms a day can help prevent many forms of cancer (Hochman, 1988; Wasowicz, 1994).
- The average diet contains 50 percent of the RDA (Pizzorno, 1996).

Zinc

- Western diets are typically zinc-deficient (Prasad, 1991; Singh et al., 1989).
- Deficiencies are especially common in children, teenagers, and pregnant women (Sanstead, 1973; Hambridge,et al. 1983).
- Sixty-eight percent of Americans do not consume the RDA of zinc (Pizzorno, 1996).

Other Trace Elements

The USDA does not survey most of the essential trace elements in the American diet. Because minerals tend to be consumed as a group in foods, rather than singly as supplements, we can assume that these other nutrients, like the minerals and trace elements listed previously are deficient in significant portions of the population.

SCIENTIFIC FLAWS IN THE USDA DIET SURVEYS

Many of the studies summarized previously are based on the diet surveys conducted by the USDA. Some are conducted by phone, like an opinion poll, and individuals are asked to recall what they have eaten in the last twenty-four hours. Others are based on three-day diet diaries. These may be the most practical survey methods, but they often provide inaccurate information. Respondents are notorious for overstating the "good" foods in their diets and understating the "bad" ones. I confront this problem every week at our clinic in Boulder, Colorado. I usually ask clients to recall what they have eaten for the last three meals. Then I ask them to keep a four-day diet diary before their next visit. Invariably, the "ideal" diet they have reported on intake is much better nutritionally than what they record in their four-day diaries. But even the diet diary rarely presents the whole picture. Clients are often on their best behavior while recording their diet, and may even fail to list items they might find embarrassing. My standard interview question after reviewing the diary is: "What do you eat when you don't eat like this?" I want to find out how they eat when they are in a hurry, or their routine is disrupted, or they are under stress, or on a special occasion. They usually mention pizza, ice cream, or bingeing on sweets. When I ask them how often they go off their routine and eat this way, it is usually as often as once a week. The USDA surveys probably follow the same pattern and are not totally reliable from a scientific point of view.

The USDA's recent data on soft drink consumption illustrate this point. According to a 1989–1991 survey of American diets, the average individual consumes about two-thirds of one soft drink a day, based on telephone polls (USDA, 1992). Another branch of the Department of Agriculture, the Economic

Research Service, records per capita consumption of foods based on sales in stores. That branch reported a 1990 per capita consumption of soft drinks at a little more than double what the diet surveys showed people actually drank (USDA, 1996). Either people are throwing away half the soft drinks they buy, or they are under-reporting consumption to USDA researchers. It makes sense to assume, then, that the actual diets of Americans are probably less nutritious than the USDA reports, and that the actual mineral status of Americans is probably worse than the statistics indicate.

CURRENT MINERAL DATA

The reports on mineral malnutrition summarized previously are based on reports from the 1980s. Current evaluations do not show the situation improving. The most recent information available from USDA food surveys shows severe mineral malnutrition for most Americans (USDA, 1997). Adult females failed to meet the RDAs for calcium, magnesium, iron, and zinc. The average adult male was deficient in magnesium and zinc. Most of the other essential trace elements are not measured in the surveys.

MEDICAL EDUCATION OF PHYSICIANS

It seems an unsolvable mystery how Surgeon General Koop, a prominent physician, could conclude in the face of the common mineral deficiencies noted previously that we have passed out of the era where malnutrition was a serious medical problem. He was in a position similar to that of the chief physician of the British navy, who ignored data proving that vitamin C could save lives. The answer may lie in the nutrition education of medical doctors.

The average physician has received only about twenty classroom hours of clinical nutrition education. Most of this takes place in basic science courses in the first years of medical school, and the percentage of nutrition-related content steadily declines in the later school years and during residency and internship training. Box 4.1 shows the findings of a 1985 National Academy of Sciences review of the nutrition education in U.S. medical schools. The classroom-hour totals include all portions of any course. Most nutrition education in medical schools comes in biochemistry, physiology, and pharmacology courses. A review of medical school curricula in 1992 shows little increased attention to clinical nutrition seven years later (Burros, 1992). Even if the situation has changed in the last five years, much time will pass before this translates into the introduction of clinical nutrition into general medical practice. Doctors who entered medical school in 1992 are, for the most part, not in practice yet. Medical doctors, despite their extensive education in anatomy, physiology, pharmacology, and conventional medical techniques, are not qualified to comment on nutrition and health, unless they have pursued studies outside their medical education. If you don't believe this, ask your doctor about the average magnesium status of Americans, and ask him or her to name five symptoms or diseases that might be associated with magnesium deficiency. You can find the answers in Chapter 16.

REGISTERED DIETICIANS

In general, conventional doctors defer questions on nutrition and diets to registered dieticians, who supervise hospital diets and patient education on nutrition. R.D.s receive significantly more nutrition education than medical doctors (see Table 4.1). The table includes basic science courses because they are

BOX 4.1

SOME FACTS ABOUT NUTRITION EDUCATION
IN U.S. MEDICAL SCHOOLS

- Fewer than one-third of medical schools have a separate nutrition course. Nutrition education overall is inadequate.
- An average of only twenty-one classroom hours is devoted to any aspect of nutrition.
- Sixty percent of schools surveyed provide less than twenty hours of nutrition instruction.
- Thirty percent teach less than ten hours.
- Only 30 percent teach more than thirty hours.
- Fifteen percent of schools do not teach recommended daily allowances for nutrients.
- More than 40 percent do not teach the role of trace minerals in nutrition.
- More than half do not teach anything about nutrient-drug interactions.
- Half do not teach anything about the relationship of diet to hypertension.
- One-third teach nothing about nutritional requirements during pregnancy and lactation.
- Half teach nothing about the changing nutritional requirements of the elderly.
- More than 20 percent teach nothing about the relationship of nutrition to cardiovascular disease.
- More than 40 percent teach nothing about the relationship of diet to gastrointestinal disease.
- More than 70 percent teach nothing about the relationship of diet to immune response.

(Source: NAS, 1985)

TABLE 4.1   CLASSROOM AND CLINIC HOURS IN NUTRITION AND COUNSELING

	Naturopathic Physician	Registered Dietician	Medical Doctor
Biochemistry and physiology	345	120	398
Basic nutrition, nutrition assessment, and interpretation	72	108	21
Diet and disease; therapeutic diets	128	72	0[a]
Counseling	150	36	0[b]
Internship	1,300[c]	900[d]	0[e]
National/state exams	yes	yes	no[f]
Totals[g]	1,995	1,236	419

(Sources: The 1987 Curricula of Bastyr College, Seattle, and National College of Naturopathic Medicine, Portland; The American Dietetic Association)

Note: Medical school hours are averages of Johns Hopkins, Mayo, Yale, and Stanford medical schools, 1987 curricula

a. Not taught in most schools

b. M.D.s receive about ninety-six hours of pharmacologically oriented psychiatric clerkship, not likely to include behaviorally oriented counseling

c. Consists of dietary evaluation or treatment of most patients

d. May be performed in a food management rather than clinical setting

e. Medical internship does not normally include training in diet and disease

f. Less than 4 percent of tests are in nutritional areas, mostly in biochemistry, physiology, and pediatrics

g. Naturopathic physicians, registered dieticians, or medical doctors may take nutrition electives above and beyond this core curriculum essential to understanding how nutrition works and counseling courses because they are essential to educating patients about dietary changes. Most of a registered dietician's nutrition education focuses on basic nutrition rather than clinical nutrition topics such as nutritional interventions in disease. Although R.D.s have a significant internship requirement, the entire internship may be spent in food management training rather than clinical nutrition. I've included the training of licensed naturopathic physicians in the chart because it's a good model for physician-level training in clinical nutrition.

A registered dietician's education is very conservative in its approach to nutritional science. Scientific evidence may be approached in several ways. The most conservative is to wait until something has been proven to be absolutely true and has been accepted by formal scientific policy-making bodies such as the National Academy of Science. Another approach is to accept a scientific hypothesis as soon as the weight of published evidence tends to support it. The second approach makes the most sense, as long as the potential toxicity of a therapy is not an issue. The American Dietetic Association, which represents R.D.s, takes the first approach. Several years ago, a representative of the ADA stated in a radio interview that the association's official opinion was that no need exists for most Americans to take vitamin or mineral supplements. This was at least a decade after the publication of the studies showing general mineral malnutrition among the American public.

MINERAL MALNUTRITION AND DISEASE

I will cover the individual minerals and their relationship to disease in detail in Chapters 5 through 25. Let's look briefly here at the consequences of the common mineral deficiencies in the foods noted in Chapter 3 and the scientific surveys summarized previously (see Tables 4.2, 4.3, and 4.4). Table 4.3 shows an increase in several chronic diseases as minerals have declined in our food. Notice that magnesium deficiency is associated with each of the illnesses. We saw in Chapter 3 that a group of plants had lost about 20 percent of their magnesium content between 1963 and 1992—the same period when the diseases in Table 4.3 increased and the USDA recorded widespread magnesium deficiencies in American diets. Figure 4.1 correlates the declining magnesium in our food supply with the increased incidence of these five magnesium-deficiency diseases. The data in Table 4.3 and Figure 4.1 could be criticized as "bad" science; I would be the first to agree that they would not pass muster in a peer-reviewed journal. One could argue that the increased incidence of the diseases could be because of more efficient reporting, and the links between magnesium deficiencies and the diseases are not ironclad by scientific standards. But to pursue this material more methodically would probably require several years of statistical research. If the trends in the graph are correct, our country is headed for serious trouble. The chart may indicate the beginnings of a mineral famine that will only get worse in the coming decades.

CONCLUSION

So far in this book we've seen how minerals moving up the food chain provide food that will prevent and cure some of the most common diseases of our society, how food processing and modern agriculture strips the soil and food of its nutrients, and the impact this can have on our health. By this point, you may already be planning to head to the health food store and pick up a vitamin and mineral supplement. In Section 3, "Getting the Minerals You Need," I'll suggest dietary changes you can make to take in more minerals, and in Chapter 29, I'll try to help you

TABLE 4.2   SOME SYMPTOMS AND ILLNESSES
            POSSIBLY CAUSED BY COMMON
            MINERAL DEFICIENCIES

Mineral	Symptoms
Calcium	Brittle nails, cramps, delusions, depression, insomnia, irritability, osteoporosis, palpitations, periodontal disease, rickets, tooth decay.
Chromium	Anxiety, fatigue, glucose intolerance, adult-onset diabetes.
Copper	Anemia, arterial damage, depression, diarrhea, fatigue, fragile bones, hair loss, hypothyroidism, weakness.
Iron	Anemia, brittle nails, confusion, constipation, depression, dizziness, fatigue, headaches, inflamed tongue, oral lesions.
Magnesium	Anxiety, confusion, heart attack, hyperactivity, insomnia, nervousness, muscular irritability, restlessness, weakness.
Selenium	Impaired growth, high cholesterol, cancer, pancreatic insufficiency, weakened immune system, liver impairment, male sterility.
Zinc	Acne, amnesia, apathy, brittle nails, delayed sexual maturity, depression, diarrhea, eczema, fatigue, growth impairment, hair loss, high cholesterol, weakened immune system, impotence, irritability, lethargy, loss of appetite, loss of sense of taste, low stomach acid, male infertility, memory impairment, night blindness, paranoia, white spots on nails, impaired wound healing.

(Source: Pizzorno, 1996)

TABLE 4.3 MINERALS GO DOWN, DISEASE GOES UP:
CHANGES IN THE RATES OF SELECTED
REPORTED CHRONIC DISEASES, 1980–1994
(PER 1,000 MEMBERS OF U.S. POPULATION)

Disease	1980	1994	% Increase	Mineral Deficiencies Associated with Disease
Heart conditions	75.40	89.47	18.67	Chromium, copper, magnesium, potassium, selenium
Chronic bronchitis	36.10	56.30	55.98	Copper, iodine, iron, magnesium, selenium, zinc
Asthma	31.20	58.48	87.44	Magnesium
Tinnitus	22.60	28.24	24.98	Calcium, magnesium, zinc
Bone deformities	84.90	124.70	46.96	Calcium, copper, fluoride, magnesium

(Sources: USDC, 1996 and Werbach, 1993)

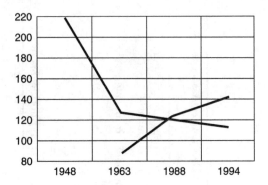

Figure 4.1   Decline in food magnesium with increase in deficiency diseases. Top line: Sums of magnesium content (in mg) in 100 g tomatoes, lettuce, cabbage, and spinach. Bottom line: Incidence of magnesium deficiency diseases, heart conditions, asthma, bronchitis, tinnitus, and orthopedic deformities (per 500 people). (Sources: Hamaker, 1982; U.S., 1989 and 1994; U.S. Department of Agriculture, 1963 and 1997; Werbach, 1993)

TABLE 4.4   MINERALS AND THE LEADING
CAUSES OF DEATH IN THE U.S.

Disease	Associated Minerals
Heart disease	Magnesium, potassium, chromium, selenium, copper
Cancer	Calcium, copper, germanium, iodine, magnesium, selenium, zinc
Stroke	Calcium, magnesium, potassium

(Source: Werbach, 1993)

sort your way through the overmarketing and occasional out-right fraud committed by the supplement industry. But first you'll learn about twenty-two minerals in detail in Section 2, "Minerals in Health and Disease." Before you start popping mineral supplements, please read that section, especially the sections on each mineral's potential toxicity. Unlike most vita-mins, "megadoses" of minerals are *never* beneficial and will in-variably cause toxicity symptoms.

MINERALS IN HEALTH AND DISEASE

IN THIS section I'll cover the effects of twenty-two minerals on human health and disease. The chapters are arranged by:

- **Function.** What we know about the role of the mineral in human physiology.
- **Recommended mineral intake.** This has two components. The first, the official U.S. recommended daily allowance (RDA), comes from the National Academy of Sciences. The second, the optimal daily intake (ODI), comes from nutrition researcher Alexander Schauss, Ph.D. Notice that the two figures are usually very close (*please* don't take megadoses of minerals) and that sometimes Schauss's recommended dosages are actually lower than the RDA.
- **Deficiency signs and symptoms.** A listing of the symptoms and illnesses that may be caused by a deficiency of the mineral.
- **Conditions treated.** These are medical conditions that physicians use the mineral to treat, either in whole-food diets or supplements. This section is for information only, and I caution you against self-medicating with mineral supplements for a disease. Minerals should

usually be taken as a group, not singly. If you are sick and do not want to take synthetic drugs, consider consulting a physician who practices nutritional medicine. I list some referral numbers in Appendix A.

- **Interactions and factors affecting absorption.** Most vitamins and minerals have complex interactions. Too much of one may cause a deficiency of another. This is one of the best reasons *not* to take individual mineral supplements, but rather to take them in a multiple vitamin and mineral supplement.

- **Toxicity and contraindications.** All minerals can be toxic if you take too high of doses for too long, and the toxic range is sometimes very close to the therapeutic range. Please consult this section before taking any mineral supplement, including those that accompany multiple vitamins. I discuss supplements in detail in Chapter 29.

- **Food sources.** I highly recommend consuming foods high in a particular mineral if you think you need more of it, rather than taking mineral supplements.

CHAPTER 5

BORON

You may already be familiar with boron in the form of the detergent Borax, with its twenty-mule team logo. Boron has long been known to be essential to plants, but was established as an essential mineral for humans in 1990. Scientists have found that boron supplements cause blood levels of calcium, magnesium, estrogen, and testosterone to rise in postmenopausal women (Nielsen et al., 1987). Its most important function in the body is maintaining healthy bones.

FUNCTION

The actual role boron plays in bone metabolism is unclear, but it seems to increase calcium absorption and utilization and reduces the amount of calcium and magnesium lost through the urine. It may act by influencing parathyroid hormone (PTH), which regulates the calcium-to-phosphorus ratio in the body. It may also help convert vitamin D into its active form, which increases the absorption of calcium from the intestines and reduces its loss through the kidneys (Block, 1979).

Boron is thought to be particularly helpful to postmenopausal women, who are at increased risk of bone loss and, consequently, osteoporosis. The mineral maintains calcium and magnesium levels in the body and also keeps levels of hormones up, particularly testosterone and estrogen, which is important to bone integrity.

Boron supplements are sometimes promoted to increase testosterone and muscle development in bodybuilders. Although boron increases testosterone levels in postmenopausal women, there is no evidence to support claims that it does so in males (Hendler, 1990).

RDA AND ODI

According to the National Research Council (a branch of the NAS), in *Recommended Daily Allowances* (10th edition, 1989), RDAs for boron have not yet been established.

Optimal Daily Intake for Boron

Males
11 to 14 years: 1.5 mg
15 to 18 years: 2.0 mg
19 and older: 2.5 mg

Females
11 to 14 years: 1.5 mg
15 to 18 years: 2.0 mg
19 to 24 years: 2.5 mg
25 and older: 3.0 mg

DEFICIENCY SIGNS AND SYMPTOMS

It is still unknown specifically what problems boron deficiency causes. The most substantial finding indicates that it may cause growth impairment. Boron deficiency may also contribute to osteoporosis. Box 5.1 shows some conditions that may be treated with increased intake of boron.

TOXICITY

Boron toxicity is rare. Daily intakes of up to 40 milligrams per day (in food) are common in some parts of the world with no known ill effects.

Acute boron toxicity, which may occur if a child eats a high quantity (more than 500 milligrams) of detergent containing boron, can cause nausea, vomiting, diarrhea, and extreme fatigue. Boron toxicity also causes a skin rash. Some of these symptoms are probably due to the loss of vitamin B_2 (riboflavin) through the urine, which occurs with acute boron overdose.

FOOD SOURCES

Boron is found in legumes, fruits, and nuts, especially those grown in arid climates. Boron content varies widely, depending

---

BOX 5.1
CONDITIONS THAT MAY BE TREATED
WITH INCREASED BORON INTAKE

Dental caries
Juvenile arthritis
Osteoporosis
Osteoarthritis

Box 5.2

Foods That Contain Boron
(Listed loosely from highest to lowest boron content)

Tomatoes	Peanuts
Pears	Almonds
Apple	Dates
Wine	Honey
Soy meal	Filbert nuts
Prunes	Seafood
Raisins	Sheep's thyroid

---

on levels in the soil. Generally, fruits and vegetables have much higher boron content than animal sources. See Box 5.2 for a list of foods that contain boron.

CHAPTER 6

CALCIUM

Calcium is the most abundant mineral in the body. In fact, it comprises as much as 2 percent of a person's total body weight. This means that if we reduced a 150-pound person to his or her essential minerals, we would find up to 3 pounds of calcium. Although 99 percent of the body's calcium is found in bones and teeth, the other 1 percent is crucial to many other essential bodily functions.

FUNCTION

Calcium combines with phosphorus to create calcium phosphate crystals, which form the bulk of the bone matrix. These crystals are incredibly light and strong, packed together within the bone in a pattern similar to the densely packed carbon crystals that form diamonds. The weight-bearing capacity of a typical bone is four times greater than an equal amount of reinforced concrete (Guiness, 1987).

Bone is a dynamic living tissue that is constantly being broken down and rebuilt. Unlike tooth enamel, which is similar in structure but cannot repair itself, bone requires a constant interplay of nutritional and hormonal factors to maintain its integrity.

The 1 percent of bodily calcium not used by bones and teeth is essential for such life processes as the passage of fluids between cell walls, clotting of blood, much of the body's enzymatic activity, release of neurotransmitters, energy production, immune function, muscle contraction, and regulation of the heartbeat. Calcium is present in the nucleus of every cell in the body, where it regulates cell reproduction and the manufacture of proteins. Calcium also adds to the stability of certain cells called *mast cells*, which are involved in immune function. When calcium is deficient, mast cells may rupture more easily, releasing chemicals known as *histamines* that cause pain and inflammation. The Krebs cycle—the body's primary mode of energy production—relies on calcium. Calcium, in conjunction with magnesium, may well be what determines our metabolic rate (Hendler, 1991).

RDA AND ODI

Recommended Daily Allowance

Infants under 6 months: 400 mg
Infants over 6 months: 600 mg
Children, 1 to 10 years: 800 mg
Males and females, 11 to 24 years: 1,200 mg
Adults, 25 years or older: 800 mg
Pregnant and lactating females: 1,200 mg
Postmenopausal women: 1,500 mg

Optimal Daily Intake

Males, 11 to 24 years: 1,000 mg
Males, 25 and older: 700 mg
Females, 11 to 24 years: 1,200 mg
Females, 25 and older: 800 mg
Postmenopausal women (51 years or older): 800 mg

DEFICIENCY SIGNS AND SYMPTOMS

Low levels of dietary calcium intake or too much phosphate (from soft drinks and processed foods) may cause the body to leach calcium from the bones to maintain blood-serum levels and/or to maintain the calcium/phosphorus balance. When bones are constantly robbed of calcium, they become weak and porous, contributing to osteoporosis.

Rickets may occur in children who have a deficiency of vitamin D, which is crucial in the metabolism of calcium. The result: bone deformities and growth retardation. In adults, this condition is known as osteomalacia, or softening of the bones.

Women and children deficient in calcium sometimes develop pica, a craving for non-food items such as clay, dirt, paint, and paste. This unusual symptom may also indicate a deficiency of zinc or iron.

Muscle spasms and leg cramps can also result from lack of sufficient calcium, as can constriction of the blood vessels, which leads to hypertension. According to Dr. Russell Marz, professor of nutrition at the National College of Naturopathic Medicine in Portland, Oregon, "periodontal disease, hyperactivity, anxiety, insomnia, and lead toxicity may also be associated with calcium deficiency" (Marz, 1997).

Box 6.1 shows some conditions that may be treated with increased intake of calcium.

INTERACTIONS AND FACTORS AFFECTING ABSORPTION

Calcium is absorbed mainly in the duodenum. The lower the pH (more acidic), the greater the absorption. At best, 30 percent of ingested calcium is absorbed. Sometimes as little as 4 percent is absorbed, especially if a person has low stomach acid,

BOX 6.1

CONDITIONS THAT MAY BE TREATED
WITH INCREASED CALCIUM INTAKE

Anxiety

Arthritis

Colon cancer (prevention)

Depression

High blood pressure

High cholesterol

Hyperactivity

Insomnia

Leg cramps

Osteoporosis

Periodontal disease

Pregnancy-induced hyper-
    tension and preeclampsia

Restless leg syndrome

a condition affecting an estimated one-third of the American population older than sixty. These people will have an extremely difficult time absorbing calcium carbonate, the most widely used calcium supplement. Most postmenopausal women should take solubilized calcium such as calcium citrate, or pre-acidified liquid calcium supplements.

Vitamin D is vital to calcium absorption from the intestinal tract and maintains blood levels essential for the proper mineralization of bone. The body makes its own vitamin D with exposure to sunlight, and the vitamin is commonly fortified in orange juice, milk, and breakfast cereals. It occurs naturally in eggs, milk, butter, and organ meats. If too much vitamin D is taken with calcium supplements, it can increase absorption to the extent that there are toxic levels of calcium in the blood.

Parathyroid hormone influences the level of calcium in the blood. It keeps calcium levels fairly stable to maintain vital bodily functions—particularly the beating of the heart. If calcium levels are too high, parathyroid hormone increases the output of calcium by the kidneys. If the calcium level is too low, it takes calcium from the bones and adds it to the blood. A parathyroid problem may cause wild fluctuation in the hormone's level, destroying the calcium balance. This can cause muscle twitches and cardiac arrhythmia.

Calcium absorption decreases with age, sedentary lifestyle, fat consumption, excess protein intake, and too much fiber. Consumption of caffeine, alcohol, sodium, and sugar increase calcium excretion in the urine. Excess phosphorus can also impair calcium absorption. Ideally, calcium and phosphoros consumption occurs in a 1:1 ratio. But many Americans eat a diet high in processed foods and soft drinks, which are high in phosphates, disrupting the balance between calcium and phosphorus. Too much phosphorus causes the body to leach calcium from the bones and, in the process, even more calcium is excreted. This is a dangerous cycle, especially since it often begins in early adolescence.

High doses of magnesium and zinc also compete with calcium for absorption. The same is true for iron, unless it is taken with vitamin C. Aluminum-containing antacids ultimately cause bone deterioration and subsequent calcium excretion. At the same time, these antacids decrease the hydrochloric acid in the stomach, thereby weakening the body's ability to absorb calcium.

Oxalates and phytates can also hinder calcium absorption. Oxalates are found in dark green leafy vegetables, especially spinach and rhubarb. Phytates are found in whole grains, seeds, nuts, and legumes. Soaking, sprouting, or fermenting the food prior to consumption can reduce phytate levels (Marz, 1997).

When taken with calcium supplements, high doses of vitamin A can stimulate bone loss. High doses of magnesium-containing supplements or medications can create toxic levels of magnesium and calcium. Potassium supplements taken with calcium increase the chance of irregular heartbeat. The drug digitalis and calcium supplements are a risky combination that may also cause irregular heartbeat (Griffith, 1986).

Diphosphates, anticonvulsants, and steroid drugs such as prednisone interfere with calcium absorption. Calcium, on the other hand, decreases the absorption of tetracycline. Birth control pills and estrogen therapies can increase calcium absorption to potentially toxic levels. If they are inappropriately prescribed, thyroid hormones, specifically T_4, have been shown to cause bone loss through excessive excretion of calcium.

TOXICITY AND CONTRAINDICATIONS

Symptoms of calcium toxicity include confusion, high blood pressure, increased sensitivity of the eyes and skin to light, increased thirst, slow or irregular heartbeat, muscle pain, nausea and vomiting, itchy skin, skin rash, and increased urination.

Calcium supplements of up to 1,500 milligrams per day are generally safe and easily tolerated. However, many factors contribute to an individual's optimum requirement, and dosages of 1,200 milligrams or less are usually sufficient to correct any deficiency. People with hyperparathyroidism, kidney disease, irregular heartbeat, and cancer should not take calcium supplements unless they are under a physician's direct supervision. Likewise, calcium supplementation may be ill-advised for people suffering from chronic constipation, colitis, or diarrhea.

Several studies have shown that some calcium supplements contain significant amounts of lead, especially those derived from dolomite or bone meal. High lead levels have been linked to low IQ and criminal behavior, as well as kidney damage and reduced red blood cell production (Murray, 1996). Refined calcium carbonate or chelated forms such as calcium citrate should be used for supplementation. Chelates are also much more easily absorbed.

BOX 6.2

FOODS HIGH IN CALCIUM (IN LOOSE ORDER OF HIGHEST TO LOWEST CALCIUM CONTENT)

Kelp	Tofu
Gruyère cheese	Oatmeal, fortified
Mozzarella cheese	Salmon, canned with
Cheddar cheese	bones
American cheese	Broccoli, cooked
Turnip greens, cooked	Vanilla ice cream
Torula yeast	Cottage cheese, 2%
Lamb's quarters, cooked	Molasses, blackstrap
Collard greens, cooked	Mustard greens, cooked
Rhubarb, cooked	Almonds
Yogurt	Beans, baked
Milk, nonfat and 2% milk	Oranges
fat	Halibut
Spinach, cooked and raw	Kale, cooked

FOOD SOURCES

The best and most readily available food sources of calcium come from dairy foods, tofu, and dark leafy greens. Sardines and canned salmon, eaten with the bones, are also good sources. See Box 6.2 for a list of foods high in calcium.

CHAPTER 7

CHROMIUM

In the 1950s, researchers found that unstable blood sugar levels in rats leveled out when the rats were fed brewer's yeast. Looking for the substance that stabilized blood sugar, scientists eventually isolated what they called the "glucose tolerance factor," or GTF. They identified chromium as the active component of GTF. Before that, chromium was considered toxic, with no role in animal or human nutrition.

FUNCTION

Chromium is vital to the function of insulin, which is required by most cells for glucose uptake. Glucose intolerance—the inability to take up glucose, the primary form of sugar the body uses—is the main symptom of diabetes. If insulin is not present, or if for some reason the cells in the body don't respond to insulin, then the cells that don't require insulin—red blood cells and those in the brain, kidneys, and eyes—overload on glucose and become damaged. Diabetics and people who have trouble controlling their blood sugar are at a much higher risk for kidney disease, blindness, and stroke. Chromium also plays a role in the metabolism of lipids (fats) and carbohydrates and appears to be related to the structural integrity of DNA and RNA, the body's genetic material.

RDA AND ODI

Recommended Daily Allowance

For males and females 11 years and older, the recommended daily allowance for chromium is 50 to 200 micrograms.

Optimal Daily Intake

Males and females, 11 to 18 years: 200 mcg
Males and females, 19 years and older: 300 mcg

DEFICIENCY SIGNS AND SYMPTOMS

As much as 90 percent of the U.S. population may be chromium deficient. As with many other minerals, food processing removes a large amount of chromium, and demineralization of farming soil in the last generation has reduced the levels in our food. In addition, high intakes of refined carbohydrates lead to an increased loss of chromium in the urine. The elderly population, pregnant women, and people who exercise regularly may be particularly at risk (Shils and Young, 1988).

The most significant symptom of chromium deficiency is impaired glucose tolerance, which can lead to diabetes mellitus and the many complications that go with that disease. Other symptoms of chromium deficiency include weight loss, peripheral neuropathy (nerve pain and/or decreased sensations in the extremities), and increased cholesterol. The most severe result of insufficient dietary chromium, observed in people who had been fed through a tube for a long period of time, was severe mental confusion associated with encephalopathy (Shils and Young, 1988).

Box 7.1 shows some conditions that may be treated with increased intake of chromium.

BOX 7.1
CONDITIONS THAT MAY BE TREATED
WITH INCREASED CHROMIUM INTAKE

Diabetes (type II)
High cholesterol
Hyperglycemia
Hypoglycemia
Obesity

INTERACTIONS AND FACTORS AFFECTING ABSORPTION

Strenuous exercise, physical trauma, and diets high in refined carbohydrates all increase the secretion of chromium through the urine. Refined sugar increases the body's need for chromium. Amino acids (the building blocks of proteins), oxalates (found in spinach and other foods), and niacin (vitamin B₃) may enhance the absorption of chromium.

TOXICITY AND CONTRAINDICATIONS

Dietary chromium has little known toxicity. However, those who are exposed to high levels of chromium dust over long periods have an increased risk of respiratory diseases, especially lung cancer (Shils and Young, 1988). There is some evidence that high doses of chromium can cause increased dream activity and reduce sleeping time. Very high doses of chromium

---

BOX 7.2

FOODS THAT CONTAIN CHROMIUM
(IN LOOSE ORDER OF HIGHEST TO
LOWEST CHROMIUM CONTENT)

Calves' liver   Cornmeal
Potatoes with skin   Brewer's yeast
Whole grain bread   Bananas
Peppers, green   Spinach
Whole grain rye bread   Cabbage
Carrots   Oranges
Apples   Blueberries

---

in animals have been associated with chromosomal damage
(Marz, 1997).

FOOD SOURCES

Brewer's yeast, oysters, liver, and potatoes contain fairly high
levels of chromium. Seafood, whole grains, cheeses, chicken,
meats, wheat bran, and fresh fruits and vegetables contain
moderate levels. Cooking in stainless steel pots may also be a
good source of chromium. This is especially true when cooking
acidic foods. The assumption is that the body can utilize
chromium incorporated into foods during preparation (Shils
and Young, 1988). See Box 7.2 for a list of foods that contain
chromium.

CHAPTER 8

COBALT

The name *cobalt* comes from the German word *kobold*, which means "goblin," and this mineral has played more than a few tricks on humans. In 1612, German miners found cobalt ore in silver mines. Thinking it contained copper, they heated the ore, releasing sickening clouds of toxic arsenic gas (F. Murray, 1995). Centuries later, in 1965, a rash of unexplained deaths occurred among heavy beer drinkers in Quebec, Nebraska, and Belgium. Cobalt had been added as a foaming agent to the beer the victims drank, and cobalt toxicity, combined with low-protein diets, was the culprit.

In 1926, doctors discovered that large doses of liver could cure pernicious anemia. When the constituent in liver responsible for the cure—vitamin B_{12}—was isolated in 1948, scientists found that cobalt was an important part of the molecule. Although cobalt can be toxic as an inorganic mineral, it is essential to life when incorporated into vitamin B_{12}.

FUNCTION

The cobalt-containing vitamin B_{12} is required for the normal production and functioning of cells. It is particularly important in the bone marrow, nervous system, and gastrointestinal tract.

RDA and ODI

Adults require approximately 1 microgram of cobalt—as a component of vitamin B_{12}—per day.

Deficiency Signs and Symptoms

There is no evidence of cobalt deficiency in humans, unless you consider cobalt's relationship to vitamin B_{12}. Pernicious anemia, which is a direct result of the body's inability to absorb vitamin B_{12}, can cause fatigue, nervous disorders, permanent nerve damage, or death. But supplementing with inorganic cobalt will not affect this disease. Pernicious anemia usually responds to vitamin B_{12} supplementation or intramuscular injection. Injection may be necessary if stomach acid is low.

Interactions and Factors Affecting Absorption

Cobalt interacts with iodine to promote normal thyroid functioning (Marz, 1997).

Toxicity and Contraindications

Cobalt is toxic and can cause heart problems, including congestive heart failure. It may also promote overproduction of red blood cells, which can increase the risk of clots and strokes.

Food Sources

Small amounts of cobalt are found in salts that are added to beer to promote foaming. Cobalt is normally ingested as a

---

BOX 8.1
FOODS THAT CONTAIN VITAMIN B$_{12}$

Clams
Fish
Meat (organs and red)
Milk
Tempeh (a fermented soy product)

---

component of vitamin B$_{12}$ (see box 8.1). Some vegetables and grains contain the mineral independent of vitamin B$_{12}$ if they are grown in cobalt-rich soils.

CHAPTER 9

COPPER

Humans have prized copper for its many uses since the Stone Age, probably as early as 8000 B.C. Ancient copper mines have been found on the island of Cyprus. In fact, the word *copper* comes from the Roman word *cuprum,* which means "Cyprean metal."

In 1925, University of Wisconsin studies showed that copper, along with iron, is necessary for hemoglobin production. In 1931, copper supplementation helped cure anemia in infants. Copper is now recognized as an essential trace element for humans and nearly every other organism.

Copper is most highly concentrated in the blood, liver, kidneys, and brain, but most other tissues and organs contain copper as well.

FUNCTION

The role of copper in the blood parallels that of iron. Copper assists in the transportation of iron and the formation of hemoglobin, the part of the red blood cell that carries oxygen from the lungs to all the cells in the body. A copper deficiency can lead to anemia, resulting in the blood's decreased capacity to carry oxygen throughout the body.

Copper contributes to the structural integrity of connective tissue throughout the body. Collagen, a protein responsible for the integrity of bone, skin, cartilage, and tendons, requires copper. Copper is also important in the structure of elastin, a connective tissue that gives elasticity to the blood vessels, lungs, and skin, allowing them to move and stretch with changes in pressure or movement.

Proper formation of the myelin sheath—the fatty substance that surrounds and protects nerve cells—depends on the presence of copper. Multiple sclerosis is a progressive degeneration of the myelin sheath.

Copper is also an antioxidant—a cofactor in the powerful enzyme, super oxide dismutase (SOD). But as with many of the antioxidants, it's possible to have too much of a good thing: Copper can also act as a free radical when taken in high dosages. This means that when copper is allowed to float freely in the blood instead of bound to its special carrier protein, ceruplasmin, it can be extremely destructive.

RDA AND ODI

Recommended Daily Allowance

Children, 10 years and younger: 1 to 1.5 mg
Males and females, 11 years and older: 1.5 to 3 mg

Optimal Daily Intake

The optimal daily intake for males and females 11 years and older is 1.5 to 4 milligrams of copper.

DEFICIENCY SIGNS AND SYMPTOMS

Copper deficiency, like iron deficiency, can lead to anemia.

Because of copper's role in the integrity of connective tissue, even a marginal copper deficiency may contribute to the formation of aneurysms, the ballooning out of the blood vessels (Murray, 1996). The aorta, the large artery that carries blood from the heart, is susceptible to aneurysm, as are some of the vessels that supply blood to the brain.

Copper deficiency can lead to impaired bone mineralization and may play a role in osteoporosis (Murray, 1996).

Because copper is essential to the formation of the myelin sheath that insulates nerves, a deficiency may also lead to damage to nerves and parts of the brain. In sheep, a deficiency of copper leads to a condition that resembles cerebral palsy (Wallach and Lan, 1994).

Box 9.1 shows some conditions that may be treated with increased copper intake.

INTERACTIONS AND FACTORS
AFFECTING ABSORPTION

Prolonged zinc supplementation can sometimes cause copper deficiency. It is always a good idea to take the two of them

---

BOX 9.1

CONDITIONS THAT MAY BE TREATED
WITH INCREASED COPPER INTAKE

Arthritis and other inflammatory conditions
Broken bones (promotes healing)
Cardiovascular disease
Impaired immune system
Osteoporosis
Vitiligo

together in a zinc-to-copper ratio of 8:1 to 10:1. In studies where healthy young men have been given high doses of zinc without copper supplementation for a considerable length of time, LDL cholesterol levels rose while HDL cholesterol fell—a pattern associated with an increased risk of heart disease.

Copper absorption is also decreased by antacids, high iron intake, vitamin C, tannins that are found in black teas, and phytates. Iron can interfere with copper absorption. Nonsteroidal anti-inflammatory drugs and penicillamine may cause copper deficiency. Long-term corticosteroid intake, which weakens connective tissue, may also cause a copper deficiency (Marz, 1997).

Copper absorption is increased by protein intake and oxalates, which are found in some green leafy vegetables, particularly spinach.

TOXICITY AND CONTRAINDICATIONS

Although copper is an antioxidant when it is attached to certain proteins and enzymes in the body, copper that is unbound in the blood is a free radical, which means it has the potential to damage cells and tissues. It may even stimulate cancer formation. High copper intake when coupled with selenium deficiency may lead to an increased risk of atherosclerosis (Schauss, 1995). So it is important not to take in too much copper; always keep any supplementation within the recommended range.

Those who are susceptible to migraine headaches should not use copper supplements. Copper may interfere with catecholamine synthesis and trigger a migraine. Sufferers of Wilson's disease, which is characterized by the accumulation of copper in the liver, eyes, and brain, and which sometimes manifests in late adolescence, should not take copper supplementation either.

Copper toxicity is often caused by drinking water that has been stored in copper pipes and may also result from cooking in copper pots. Symptoms of copper toxicity are poor memory, depression, insomnia, and joint and muscle pain. Some people experience symptoms similar to zinc toxicity, including nausea and vomiting, when they supplement with copper. Long-term copper supplementation may cause cirrhosis of the liver. Large doses of vitamin C may lower serum copper levels.

FOOD SOURCES

Copper is found in many foods. It is particularly rich in shellfish, especially oysters. Organ meats, legumes, sesame seeds, nuts, yeast, mushrooms, and dried fruit are also good sources. See Box 9.2 for a list of foods containing copper.

BOX 9.2

FOODS HIGH IN COPPER (IN LOOSE ORDER FROM HIGHEST TO LOWEST COPPER CONTENT)

Beef liver	Bananas
Millet	Sunflower seeds
Rye	Peanuts
Cocoa powder	Mushrooms
Beans	Halibut
Prunes	Tofu, firm
Brazil nuts	Wheat germ
Barley	Pinto beans
Cashews	Apricots
Chicken, light meat	Almonds
Peas	Sesame seeds, unhulled
Pecans	Whole wheat flour
Molasses, blackstrap	

CHAPTER 10

FLUORIDE

In the 1940s, public health officials noted that people living in certain parts of the country developed brown stains on their teeth. Despite the stains, these people had significantly lower levels of tooth decay. The common factor among the areas was high levels of fluoride in the drinking water. At the time fluoride had been added in large quantities to kill bacteria, rats, and insects. Soon afterward, researchers discovered that smaller amounts of fluoride in the water could decrease tooth decay without causing the unappealing side effect of brown mottling of the teeth. The fluoridation of drinking water became national public policy.

FUNCTION

Although fluoride is a normal component of calcified tissue, it is not considered an essential mineral for humans. It appears to stimulate osteoblasts (young bone cells) to increase collagen synthesis and deposit calcium. Fluoride combines with calcium to give bones and teeth their density. In teeth, fluoride enhances and hardens the enamel to decrease the incidence of cavities (Hendler, 1990); it also fights bacteria associated with increased tooth decay. In 1988, the American Institute for Dental Research studied forty thousand U.S. children between the ages of

5 and 17 years and found a 36 percent decrease in the overall number of cavities, possibly due to fluoridation of the drinking water (Hendler, 1990).

RDA AND ODI

No recommended daily allowance or optimal daily intake for fluoride has been established, but 1.5 to 4 milligrams per day should be sufficient. Water contains about 1 milligram per liter, or 1 part per million. More than 4 parts per million of fluoride is considered toxic.

DEFICIENCY SIGNS AND SYMPTOMS

Increased tooth decay and cavity formation are the only symptoms associated with a diet low in fluoride. Intake of fluoride will protect teeth from future decay.

INTERACTIONS AND FACTORS AFFECTING ABSORPTION

Calcium can be used as an antidote for fluoride toxicity in the event that large quantities of mouthwash or toothpaste with fluoride are inadvertently swallowed.

TOXICITY AND CONTRAINDICATIONS

Fluoride can be very toxic. Chronic ingestion of 2.5 parts per million or more in children will strengthen their teeth and bones, but will also cause permanent mottling of teeth. At 3 to 5 parts per million, toxic effects have resulted in cattle in the form of weakness, loss of appetite, and gastroenteritis. Human gastroenteritis has been associated with fluoride ingestion at slightly higher levels. Other symptoms of long-term exposure (ingestion of 8 parts per million per day over 35 years) include skeletal abnormalities including osteoporosis and/or osteomalacia, calcification of tendons and ligaments, as well as development of bone spurs.

Signs and symptoms of acute fluoride toxicity include cramping, nausea, diarrhea, and joint pain.

Long-term exposure to high levels of fluoride (20 to 80 milligrams per day) can lead to a condition known as skeletal fluorisis, which is a hardening of the bones accompanied by arthritic pain, stiffness, and nerve damage, in some cases leading to paralysis. There is some evidence that fluoride increases the risk of certain types of oral, bone, thyroid, and liver cancer in rats (Wallach and Lan, 1994, and Griffiths, 1990).

BOX 10.1

FOODS THAT CONTAIN FLUORIDE
(IN LOOSE ORDER FROM HIGHEST TO
LOWEST FLUORIDE CONTENT)

Mackerel	Lettuce	Apples
Tea	Wine	Chicken
Coffee	Sardines	Milk, whole
Rice	Salmon	Eggs
Buckwheat	Potatoes	Kale
Soybeans	Cod	Grapefruit
Spinach	Shrimp	Oatmeal
Onions	Beef	Corn

(Source: Gordenoff and Member, 1962)

FOOD SOURCES

Fluoride can be found in seafood, black tea, toothpaste, and fluoridated water. Cooking with Teflon pans may also contribute to fluoride levels (Marz, 1997). See Box 10.1 for a list of foods containing fluoride.

CHAPTER 11

GERMANIUM

Germanium has been touted as a tissue oxygenator, although its necessary role in the human body has not yet been proven. In fact, no requirement for germanium in any organism has been demonstrated (Schauss, 1995).

FUNCTIONS

Although germanium has no proven biological function in the human body, a synthetic organic compound of germanium known as Ge-132 is reputed to cure a number of chronic diseases and is widely sold in health food stores. It may increase our cellular oxygen uptake, although these claims have yet to be proven. According to Dr. Kazuhiko Asai, who isolated organic germanium as a healing substance, it is "capable of eliminating harmful substances causing disease in the body" (Asai, 1980). In addition, germanium may be used by the thyroid, indicating a possible role in the function of thyroid hormones (Marz, 1997).

Animal studies have shown that germanium may bolster the immune system and act as an anticancer agent. Test tube studies on germanium's inhibiting effect on the reproduction of the human immunodeficiency virus (HIV) look promising (Hendler, 1990).

BOX 11.1
FOODS THAT CONTAIN GERMANIUM

Beans
Chlorella
Garlic
Ginseng
Pearl barley
Shiitake mushrooms
Tuna
Water chestnuts

RDA AND ODI

There is little reliable information on recommended intake for germanium, but we probably ingest about 1.5 milligrams per day with a typical American diet. Doses exceeding 30 milligrams per day (7.5 milligrams per day for children) are not recommended (Schauss, 1995).

DEFICIENCY SIGNS AND SYMPTOMS

There is no deficiency syndrome associated with germanium.

TOXICITY AND CONTRAINDICATIONS

Side effects associated with germanium supplementation have been limited mostly to skin irritation and mild diarrhea, but serious kidney damage is also a risk. At least twenty cases of germanium-induced kidney toxicity have been reported in scientific articles. The suspected cause is inorganic germanium contaminants in supposedly "organic" Ge-132 supplements (Schauss, 1991, and Matsusaka et al., 1988).

FOOD SOURCES

See Box 11.1 for food sources rich in germanium.

CHAPTER 12

THE
ELECTROLYTES:
POTASSIUM,
SODIUM, AND
CHLORIDE

Electrolytes are chemicals that have an electrical charge on them, making them capable of conducting electricity. They are either positive—like sodium, potassium, calcium, and others—or negative, like chloride and phosphate. Potassium, sodium, and chloride are the most prominent of the electrolytes, and they interact to regulate a number of key physiological functions.

FUNCTIONS

Electrolytes control osmosis, the movement of water from outside of the cell through the membrane and into the cell; they help maintain the acid-base balance required for normal cellular activity; and they carry electrical currents that travel down nerves—allowing muscles to contract—and release some hormones and neurotransmitters along the way.

Potassium and sodium allow the electrical activity of the human body to occur. This includes the heartbeat, nervous impulses, muscle contractions, and much more. Potassium collects within the cell, while sodium remains outside in the extracellular fluid. These two minerals, along with negatively charged chloride and phosphate, set up a *potential*, a difference between the inside and the outside of the cell—much like a battery—that allows the electrical energy to occur. Potassium also acts as a catalyst in carbohydrate and protein metabolism.

The electrolytes also help the body adapt to stress. When startled, the human body quickly goes into its "fight-or-flight" state in order to adapt to a potentially life-threatening stress. Blood rushes to the skeletal muscles, heart, brain, and lungs. Glucose, the sugar used as fuel, floods into the blood and muscles to give us strength to run away or to fight. Potassium is excreted into the urine, while sodium is spared to maintain blood pressure and volume. This is important so that, if injured, we don't collapse in shock.

However, our systems aren't designed for the prolonged periods of stress that work, traffic, finances, and relationships bring. Chronic stress depletes our bodily stores of numerous precious nutrients, and potassium is particularly at risk.

Chloride is also used to form hydrochloric acid, which is crucial to the digestion of proteins and assists in the absorption of many nutrients, including calcium, iron, and vitamin B_{12}.

RDA AND ODI

Recommended Daily Allowance

Although there is no actual RDA for potassium, 1,600 milligrams a day is needed to maintain bodily stores and normal concentration in the blood and bodily fluids. Males and females 11 and older should have 2 grams of potassium a day in their diet. It has been found that if a person eats just one serving of fruit or vegetable per day (not even the recommended three), he or she reduces the risk of heart disease and stroke by 40 percent (Hendler, 1990).

Optimal Daily Intake

Males and Females
11 to 14 years: 2 g
15 to 18 years: 2.5 g
19 years and older: 3 g

DEFICIENCY SIGNS AND SYMPTOMS

Potassium deficiency is a serious problem because it can interfere with the normal rhythm of the heart and trigger a heart attack. An early symptom of inadequate potassium intake is muscle weakness. Cramping, shallow breathing, fatigue, nausea, vomiting, confusion, and increased urination are also possible symptoms. Both high blood pressure and cancer may be treated with increased potassium intake.

Sodium deficiency is very rare in Western culture. However, sodium loss can result from excessive perspiration, burns, vomiting, and diarrhea. Symptoms of sodium deficiency are muscle weakness, dizziness, headaches, decreased blood pressure, increased heart rate, and shock. In severe cases it can lead to mental confusion, stupor, and even coma (Tortora, 1994).

Chloride deficiency is also uncommon. However, it can result from vomiting, diarrhea, and the use of certain diuretics. Symptoms are muscle spasms, decreased respiration, and, in extreme cases, coma.

INTERACTIONS AND FACTORS AFFECTING ABSORPTION

Magnesium helps maintain intracellular levels of potassium, while caffeine, diuretics, and laxatives increase urinary excretion of potassium.

Lithium increases the excretion of sodium. People who are taking prescription lithium drugs should not restrict their sodium intake as it can have dangerous consequences.

High sodium in general increases the excretion of potassium and vice versa.

TOXICITY AND CONTRAINDICATIONS

Potassium

Again, potassium has an optimal range within the body. Exceeding or dropping too far below that range can be potentially lethal since it can affect the rhythm of the heart and potentially cause a heart attack. People with kidney damage and hypertension—who should be under a physician's care—must maintain special watch over their potassium levels.

Early signs of potassium toxicity are nausea and diarrhea. More serious symptoms include an irregular heartbeat, paralysis of the arms and legs, a sudden drop in blood pressure, convulsions, and even coma or cardiac arrest (Griffith, 1988).

Sodium

Water loss or deprivation and high dietary sodium intake can lead to general dehydration and symptoms of sodium toxicity such as intense thirst, fatigue, agitation, and, in acute cases, coma. Too much sodium increases the requirement for potassium and throws off the sodium/potassium balance. Prolonged sodium/potassium imbalance is associated with hypertension, increased incidence of kidney stones, osteoporosis, and congestive heart failure.

FOOD SOURCES

Potassium is primarily found in fruits and vegetables. Bananas and cantaloupe are particularly rich sources. See Box 12.1 for a list of good sources of potassium.

BOX 12.1
FOODS THAT CONTAIN POTASSIUM
(IN LOOSE ORDER FROM HIGHEST TO LOWEST POTASSIUM CONTENT)

Avocados	Broccoli
Apricots, dried	Tomatoes
Potatoes	Pinto beans
Cantaloupe	Bananas
Lima beans	Milk
Parsnips	Sweet potatoes
Raisins	Salmon
Sardines	Beans, great northern
Flounder	Cod, baked
Orange juice	Liver, beef
Soybeans	Artichokes
Squash, winter	Peaches

The major source for chloride is sodium chloride, or table salt, which is often added as a flavoring and preservative to many canned and processed foods. Processed foods also contain other forms of sodium, including sodium nitrate, monosodium glutamate (MSG), sodium benzoate, sodium bicarbonate (baking soda), and sodium phosphate. Sodium is also found naturally in dairy products, meats, fish, and some vegetables. There are considerable quantities of sodium in many drugs including aspirin, antacids, and some antibiotics.

Box 12.2 provides a list of high-sodium foods—these are the ones to avoid in favor of fresh fruit and vegetables. A single serving of most vegetables contains less than 20 milligrams of sodium. In contrast, the foods in Box 12.2 contain 500 or more

---

BOX 12.2

FOODS HIGH IN SODIUM (IN ORDER OF
HIGHEST TO LOWEST SODIUM CONTENT)

Lox (smoked salmon)	Feta cheese
Anchovy paste	McDonald's Egg
Soy sauce	McMuffin
American cheese	Tortilla chips
McDonald's Quarter-	Corned beef
pounder with Cheese	Fried chicken
Baking soda	Ham
Bologna	Canadian bacon
Corn chips	Cheddar cheese

TABLE 12.1   FOOD LABELING AND
SODIUM CONTENT

Label	Definition
Sodium-free	Less than 5 mg per standard serving and does not contain any sodium chloride
Very low sodium	35 mg or less per serving
Low sodium	140 mg or less per serving
Reduced sodium	At least 25% less sodium per serving than the regular recipe
Light in sodium	50% less sodium per serving than in the regular recipe
Unsalted	No added salt during processing (unlike the standard, salted recipe, as in nuts, for example)
Lightly salted	50% less added sodium than normal

milligrams of sodium per serving. Table 12.1 provides definitions of common sodium-related food labeling, to help you when you shop for low-sodium items.

CHAPTER 13

IODINE

In ancient China as early as 3000 B.C., burnt sponges and seaweed were used to treat goiter, a swelling of the thyroid gland often caused by iodine deficiency. In Greece nearly twenty-five hundred years later, Hippocrates described using the same treatment.

The element iodine was discovered by French chemist Bernard Courtois in the nineteenth century. As he was touring a gun powder factory, he noticed purple vapors rising from the heating vats where gunpowder was being prepared. Seaweed ash was being used as a source of sodium carbonate. Upon further investigation, Courtois discovered that the seaweed ash contained another mineral that was responsible for the violet vapors. Courtois used the Greek word, *iodes*, which means violet, to name this new mineral. Iodine was the second mineral established as essential to human life, after iron in the previous century.

While iodine is plentiful in the oceans and in foods derived from the sea, it is thinly and unevenly distributed in the earth's crust. Consequently, many people — particularly those who live in mountainous regions or in the middle of the continent — develop iodine deficiencies. Despite the introduction of iodized salt in 1924 and its general use in developed countries, iodine deficiency remains as one of the most prevalent mineral deficiencies, affecting more than 500 million people worldwide (Murray, 1995).

FUNCTION

Almost half of the body's iodine resides in the thyroid gland. Thyroid hormones control energy metabolism as well as body temperature, reproduction, and growth. No other known functions of iodine have been proven. However, it does seem to concentrate in the gastric mucosa (the tissue that lines the stomach), salivary glands, and lactating mammary glands. Evidence suggests that breast tissue requires elemental iron to modulate estrogen.

RDA AND ODI

Recommended Daily Allowance

Infants to 6 months: 40 mcg
Infants, 6 to 12 months: 50 mcg
Toddlers, 1 to 3 years: 70 mcg
Children, 4 to 6 years: 90 mcg
Children, 7 to 10 years: 120 mcg
Males and females, 11 years and older: 150 mcg
Pregnant women: 175 mcg
Lactating women: 200 mcg

Optimal Daily Intake

The optimal daily intake of iodine for adults is 150 micrograms.

DEFICIENCY SIGNS AND SYMPTOMS

The thyroid gland is located in the neck. Because iodine is an important component of thyroid hormones, the thyroid attempts to compensate for a lack of iodine by increasing the manufacture and output of thyroid hormones. This causes the gland to swell, creating a goiter. Females require higher iodine levels during periods such as puberty and pregnancy when the metabolic rate is high, and are more prone to goiter than men.

Some goiters are not due to a simple iodine deficiency. Overactivity of the thyroid gland, called hyperthyroidism, is sometimes accompanied by goiterous swelling. This condition, known as Graves' disease, can lead to a massive increase in metabolism and can be life-threatening. Cancer of the thyroid gland can also cause swelling in the neck. A number of pharmaceutical drugs may also induce goiter.

Hypothyroidism, decreased levels of thyroid hormones, can cause sluggishness, slowed heart rate, increased cholesterol, weight gain, constipation, and an increased need for sleep. While small amounts of iodine may correct a state of low thyroid function, large amounts can actually suppress the thyroid and further exacerbate the problem.

Babies of iodine-deficient mothers can develop a condition known as *cretinism*, which can lead to physical and mental retardation if it is left untreated. In countries where iodine deficiency is common, cretinism is endemic, with widespread incidence of deaf-mutism, paralysis, and mental retardation (Shils and Young, 1988).

Box 13.1 shows some conditions that may be treated with increased iodine intake.

INTERACTIONS AND FACTORS AFFECTING ABSORPTION

Goitrogens occur naturally in foods and block absorption or utilization of iodine. Goitrogenic foods include cabbage, turnips, rapeseeds, peanuts, cassava melon, and soybeans. Cooking these

---

BOX 13.1

CONDITIONS THAT MAY BE TREATED
WITH INCREASED IODINE INTAKE

Fibrocystic breast disease
Goiter (some types)
Immunodeficiency
Radiation toxicity (prevention)

---

foods generally inactivates the goitrogens. A number of pharmaceutical drugs are also goitrogenic.

TOXICITY AND CONTRAINDICATIONS

Iodine is a safe mineral in a wide range of doses, but it is important not to overdo it because it can suppress the thyroid and cause symptoms of hypothyroidism. And although iodine is used to treat goiter, too much of it can *cause* a goiter as well (Griffith, 1988).

The first signs that you are overdoing iodine could include a rash, depression, aggravation of acne, or nausea. Headaches, tiredness, weakness, or a sensation of heaviness are also signs of excess iodine. Other iodine-related problems are numbness and tingling, swelling of the salivary glands, a metallic taste in the mouth, and salivation. If any of these symptoms occur while you are taking iodine, stop taking it immediately.

Do not take iodine supplements if you are on lithium carbonate, which is given to treat bipolar disorder (manic depression). The lithium already decreases the activity of the thyroid

---

BOX 13.2

FOODS THAT CONTAIN IODINE

Cod	Herring
Dulse	Kelp
Haddock	Sardines
Halibut	Shrimp

---

and taking an iodine supplement can further aggravate that side effect (Griffith, 1988).

FOOD SOURCES

Seafood is a rich source of iodine (see Box 13.2). Iodophores, which are used as antiseptics in the dairy industry, and iodized salt are the main sources of iodine in most diets. Iodine levels are extremely variable in foods and drinking water. Iodine content in fruits and vegetables depends on the soil and fertilizer the produce is grown in, and how it is processed.

CHAPTER 14

IRON

Iron was once considered the metal of the heavens, and scientists believe that early prized samples of iron probably came from meteors. The ancient Greeks used iron as a health tonic. They would soak their iron swords in hot water and then use the iron-enriched water to treat anemia.

Most of the iron in the human body resides in the red blood cells in the form of hemoglobin, which carries oxygen from the lungs to cells throughout the body. Hemoglobin also transports carbon dioxide from the cells back to the lungs, where the carbon dioxide is exhaled.

Not everyone needs extra iron. The body very efficiently recycles and uses the iron it has. Unless you lose it through chronic bleeding or a high metabolic state—as in pregnancy or childhood—you probably can get all the iron you need from the food you eat.

FUNCTION

Most of the body's iron is used to make hemoglobin. Iron is also important in energy release, immune function, and cholesterol metabolism. Myoglobin, which is present in muscles, also contains iron. It helps deliver oxygen and, consequently, energy to muscles when they are working hard.

Iron is stored in the liver, spleen, and bone marrow in the form of ferritin, which is used to make more hemoglobin when the need arises. Most of the iron in the body is recycled when red blood cells die. Low levels of ferritin in the blood indicate long-term iron deficiency.

Iron works in the immune system to fight invading bacteria and viruses. It also assists with detoxification in the liver. Important in the growth process, iron is a constituent in many enzymes and proteins in the body, including the synthesis of DNA (Griffith, 1986).

RDA AND ODI

Recommended Daily Allowances

Children
Infants to 6 months: 10 mg
6 to 12 months: 15 mg
1 to 3 years: 15 mg
4 to 10 years: 10 mg

Males
11 to 18 years: 12 mg
19 years and older: 10 mg

Females
11 years and older: 15 mg
Pregnant: 30 to 60 mg
Lactating: 30 to 60 mg

Optimal Daily Intake

Males
11 to 18 years: 15 mg
18 years and older: 20 mg

Females
11 to 18 years: 20 mg
18 to 50 years: 22 mg
50 years and older: 20 mg

DEFICIENCY SIGNS AND SYMPTOMS

Iron deficiency is the most common cause of anemia. Young boys ages six to eight and young women in their teens are most vulnerable to deficiency because of their rapid growth rates. For young women, blood lost during menstruation is also a factor. People who suffer from chronic blood loss—such as those with gastrointestinal bleeding—are similarly at risk. Iron deficiency can also *cause* excessive bleeding (Taymore et al., 1964).

The symptoms of iron-deficiency anemia include headaches, shortness of breath, weakness, fatigue, heart palpitations, intolerance to cold, and a sore tongue. As the iron deficiency becomes more severe, epithelial tissues are affected, especially the tongue, nails, mouth, and stomach. Fingernails become thin, flat, and even severely spoon shaped. Symptoms affecting the tongue include atrophy of the tongue papillae, burning, redness, and, in severe cases, a completely smooth and waxy appearance.

Iron deficiency in infants and young children is associated with slow mental and motor development, even after the problem has been corrected. Iron-deficiency in infants may also cause behavioral problems such as an increased tendency to be unhappy, tired, and tense during medical examinations. An infant is especially vulnerable during the second six months of life; any problems caused by iron deficiency may become permanent (Lozoff, 1991).

Pica, a rare condition typically affecting small children and women where one craves nonfood items such as laundry starch, dirt, chalk, or ashes, can be caused by an iron deficiency. Pica can also be caused by magnesium and calcium deficiencies.

Box 14.1 shows some conditions that may be treated with increased iron intake.

INTERACTIONS AND FACTORS AFFECTING ABSORPTION

Iron derived from animal sources is known as *heme* iron. It is much more readily absorbed than iron from nonanimal sources, which is called *non-heme* iron. The body absorbs up to 35 percent of iron from heme sources, but it can absorb only up to 2.9 percent of non-heme iron (Murray, 1996). In addition, heme iron does not seem to cause the same unpleasant side effects — nausea, flatulence, and diarrhea — as non-heme iron (Krause and Mahan, 1984). Growth phases, menstruation, and pregnancy also affect iron absorption.

Vitamin C and stomach acid enhance the absorption of iron, particularly from non-heme sources. When the body increases production of hemoglobin, such as after a trauma or surgery, or when a person suffers from anemia, absorption increases as well. The presence of calcium, except in very high doses, can also increase absorption.

BOX 14.1

CONDITIONS THAT MAY BE TREATED
WITH INCREASED IRON INTAKE

Anemia
Menorrhagia (excessive menstrual bleeding)
Restless Leg Syndrome

Phosphates (found in eggs, cheese, and milk), oxalates, phytates, and tannins (found in black teas, bran, and coffee) inhibit iron absorption. Vitamin E and high zinc levels decrease iron absorption by binding iron in the gut.

TOXICITY AND CONTRAINDICATIONS

Unless you are at risk for iron-deficiency anemia or have been tested to indicate that you need it, it is best not to supplement with iron. This is especially true if you have an active inflammation or infection. Although iron is used by the immune system to fight certain pathogens—bacteria, viruses, parasites, and fungi—the mineral can in fact feed other bacteria. Furthermore, it is much harder to correct an iron abundance than it is a deficiency. The body tends to stockpile iron, which can trigger an increasingly common condition known as hemachromatosis. Hemachromatosis was once thought to be rare, but is now showing up in many people. The body stores iron in vital organs such as the liver, pancreas, and heart, carrying the potential to do extensive damage. Symptoms of hemachromatosis include weight loss, weakness, change in skin color, abdominal pain, decreased sex drive, and onset of diabetes.

Research has found that there may be an increased risk of infections, certain types of cancer, and heart disease in people who have elevated iron levels. As a free radical, iron can cause damage to tissue, including low-density lipoproteins—the "bad" form of cholesterol—which, when damaged, is thought to increase the risk of atherosclerosis.

People who suffer from rheumatoid arthritis should not take supplemental iron. As a free radical, iron may contribute to the inflammation and swelling.

Some people simply do not tolerate iron supplements well and may develop side effects such as heartburn, nausea, constipation, or diarrhea.

BOX 14.2

FOODS THAT CONTAIN IRON (IN LOOSE ORDER
OF HIGHEST TO LOWEST IRON CONTENT)

Beef liver	Beef
Tuna	Collard greens
Blackstrap molasses	Roast beef
Pumpkin	Beet greens
Oysters	Lima beans
Oatmeal	Brewer's yeast
Tofu	Figs
Cocoa powder	Sunflower seeds
Swiss chard	Raisins
Peas	Mustard greens

Iron poisoning is the most common accidental poisoning in young children, and it can be fatal. Some iron tablets are small, round pills coated with sugar that look like candy. In 1991, more than 5,000 children overdosed on iron pills, and nine of them died. Severe iron poisoning can cause damage to the intestinal lining, liver failure, nausea, vomiting, and death (Murray, 1995). It is extremely important to keep all iron supplements out of the reach of children.

FOOD SOURCES

Animal sources provide iron in the form most easily absorbed by the body. Some plant sources, such as spinach, also have high iron content, but it is not easily absorbed. A significant amount of iron, perhaps even toxic levels, can be "added" to food by cooking it in cast-iron pots and pans, which should be avoided.

See Box 14.2 for a list of good dietary sources of iron.

CHAPTER 15

LITHIUM

Since 1951, each succeeding generation of Americans has had a nearly twofold increase in the incidence of clinical depression. The average age of early-onset depression continues to drop, and it is now common to see these signs in adolescents. Psychiatrists contend that depression is primarily a psychological disorder stemming from unexpressed anger and grief, a lack of self-worth, and a general sense of impotence and ineffectiveness, but as we see in Table 25.1, depression is associated with multiple mineral and vitamin deficiencies, including lithium.

Depression is most often clinically treated with large doses of lithium (Wallach and Lan, 1994). It also appears to have biological effects in the tiny doses available in food.

FUNCTION

Lithium is stored in the pituitary, ovaries, thyroid, and adrenal glands. It may play a role in fertility and in cellular uptake of glucose (Marz, 1997, and Birch, 1978).

Lithium may help prevent atherosclerosis in people who respond to sodium restriction. Lithium can displace sodium because of its similar chemical composition (Anke et al., 1981, and Voors et al., 1971).

In several studies, researchers have found a correlation between low water levels of lithium and increased violent crime and behavior. These results suggest that lithium may help inhibit certain violent impulses. Similarly, problems with addictions appear to occur less often in areas with high levels of lithium in drinking water (Frieden, 1984).

RDA and ODI

No recommended daily allowance for lithium has been established. Schauss's optimal daily intake, however, is between 2 and 3 milligrams of lithium per day.

Deficiency Signs and Symptoms

Animals placed on a lithium-deficient diet exhibited a decreased growth rate and less overall fertility. This suggests that lithium may be an essential nutrient.

As we've already discussed, manic depression can be relieved by an increased intake of lithium.

Interactions and Factors Affecting Absorption

Lithium displaces sodium in the body. To avoid a sodium deficiency, do not restrict your intake of salt if you are taking lithium carbonate.

There is some evidence to suggest that an accumulation of the mineral vanadium is associated with bipolar disorder. Vanadium appears in higher levels in the hair of people who are diagnosed with manic depression. It is thought that lithium may work by counteracting the effects of vanadium (Schauss, 1995).

BOX 15.1
FOODS THAT CONTAIN LITHIUM

Beef liver	Legumes
Eggplant	Peppers
Grains	Potatoes
Leafy green vegeta-	Seafood
bles	Tomatoes

TOXICITY AND CONTRAINDICATIONS

Normal nutritional intake of 5 to 10 milligrams per day rarely causes lithium toxicity. However, pregnant or lactating women should not take lithium.

Heart or kidney disease can induce lithium toxicity, which can cause dehydration and sodium depletion. A physician should regularly monitor blood lithium levels of those taking the mineral therapeutically. The large doses used for manic depression treatment can cause a wide variety of unpleasant side effects.

FOOD SOURCES

"Hard" water provides a significant source of lithium. Artesian wells and mineral springs are purportedly richer in lithium than other sources of drinking water. Foods from the night shade family are also rich in the mineral. See Box 15.1 for a list of dietary sources of lithium.

CHAPTER 16

MAGNESIUM

All life came from the sea. The chemical composition of our cells contains the code of the sea just as children contain genetic information they received from their parents. We require the balance of minerals that existed in the sea to maintain optimum health. The primordial sea contained high quantities of magnesium, among other minerals. Similarly, the waters of our cells are rich in magnesium.

Magnesium is a major factor in our bodies, comprising about 0.05 percent of our body weight. Magnesium deficiency is the most common deficiency in the U.S. diet.

FUNCTIONS

Magnesium is involved in the activation of at least three hundred different enzymes and body chemicals. It activates the B vitamins and plays a role in protein synthesis, muscle excitability, and energy release. It is mainly found in the mitochondria, the energy centers of cells. Magnesium regulates the absorption of calcium and adds to the integrity of the bones and teeth. Deficiency of magnesium can lead to bone abnormalities including brittle bones and osteoporosis. The parathyroid gland, which regulates blood calcium levels, also needs magnesium to function normally (Marz, 1997).

Concentrated eighteen times greater in the heart muscle than in the bloodstream, magnesium regulates the heart's ability to beat. It decreases blood coagulation and acts as a calcium channel blocker, helping the heart pump more effectively. In addition, magnesium has a relaxing effect on smooth muscle and possibly blood vessels. Uterine relaxation in response to magnesium may lessen the intensity of menstrual cramps. Magnesium is vital to energy production on the cellular level. It is also required for the proper transmission of nerve impulses (Marz, 1997).

RDA AND ODI

Recommended Daily Allowance

Children
250 mg

Males
11 to 14 years: 270 mg
15 to 18 years: 400 mg
19 years and older: 350 mg

Females
11 to 14 years: 280 mg
15 to 18 years: 300 mg
19 years and older: 280 mg
Lactating women: 410–425 mg

Optimal Daily Intake

Males
11 to 14 years: 300 mg
15 to 18 years: 500 mg

19 to 50 years: 500 mg
51 years and older: 600 mg

Females
11 to 14 years: 300 mg
15 to 18 years: 400 mg
19 to 50 years: 450 mg
51 years and older: 550 mg

DEFICIENCY SIGNS AND SYMPTOMS

Magnesium deficiency is often overlooked because it is not associated with any specific syndromes. Muscle weakness, loss of appetite, nausea, vomiting, diarrhea, fatigue, nervousness, and irritability can all be early signs of magnesium deficiency. More serious symptoms include muscle spasms and seizures.

Magnesium is intimately related to the regulation of calcium. When magnesium is low, blood becomes saturated with calcium, which it often deposits in the muscles or kidneys. This can lead to kidney stones.

There is evidence that magnesium deficiency may play a critical role in many heart ailments. When Dr. Alexander Heggtveit, professor of pathology at the University of Ottawa in Canada, examined the victims of fatal heart attacks and found that certain portions of the heart contained up to 42 percent less magnesium than heart muscle from individuals who died of other causes.

Magnesium deficiency can occur after prolonged vomiting or diarrhea, with long-term diuretic and or laxative use, and after alcohol abuse. A high intake of calcium can increase excessive magnesium excretion, leading to problems such as nervousness, irritability, and tremors. Deficiency can also cause muscle contraction and may contribute to hallucinations in people going through alcohol withdrawal (Griffith, 1988).

The elderly population is especially at risk for magnesium deficiency due to poor absorption, excess calcium supplementation, and drug interactions.

Box 16.1 shows some conditions that may be treated with increased magnesium intake.

INTERACTIONS AND FACTORS AFFECTING ABSORPTION

Many factors regulate magnesium absorption. Generally, as the level of calcium intake goes down, the level of magnesium absorption goes up. A significant amount of magnesium goes to the stomach for hydrochloric acid production. High intakes of calcium, protein, vitamin D, and alcohol all increase the magnesium requirement. Caffeine, phosphorus, sugar, high sodium, thiazide diuretics, and alcohol all increase the loss of magnesium through the urine. Magnesium supplementation can compete with calcium for uptake and can thus exacerbate a calcium deficiency. This can be eliminated by taking the two minerals in balanced doses.

BOX 16.1

CONDITIONS THAT MAY BE TREATED WITH INCREASED MAGNESIUM INTAKE

Cardiovascular disease
Chronic fatigue syndrome
Kidney stones (prevention)
Muscle cramps
Preeclampsia (during pregnancy)

BOX 16.2
FOODS THAT CONTAIN MAGNESIUM
(IN LOOSE ORDER OF HIGHEST TO LOWEST
MAGNESIUM CONTENT)

Fermented soy products	Beet greens
	Oats
Peanuts	Avocados
Leafy green vege-	Black-eyed peas
tables	Baked potatoes with
Seeds	skin
Buckwheat flour	Almonds
Walnuts	Millet
Whole wheat flour	Brown rice
Bananas	Blackstrap molasses

Magnesium absorption increases in the presence of lactose (the sugar found in milk), vitamin D, and probably acid. On a cellular level, vitamin B_6 can help the cells take in magnesium.

TOXICITY AND CONTRAINDICATIONS

Generally, the incidence of magnesium toxicity as a result of oral supplementation is low. Excess magnesium is usually excreted quickly by the onset of diarrhea. However, because it is present in many over-the-counter medications, consumers should be aware of the possibility of magnesium toxicity. This is especially true for people who take larger than the recommended amounts of antacids and laxatives. Fourteen deaths from magnesium toxicity have occurred in the United States over the past two decades (Griffith, 1988).

FOOD SOURCES

Magnesium is plentiful in whole foods. The best sources of magnesium are fermented soy products, legumes, nuts, seeds, and leafy green vegetables. See Box 16.2 for more food sources of magnesium.

CHAPTER 17

MANGANESE

Manganese is essential to all known living organisms. Before the earth's atmosphere contained oxygen, when life on earth was just beginning, algae was able to derive oxygen from water and the energy of the sun. Manganese is thought to have made this reaction possible (Hendler, 1990).

Manganese was recognized and isolated as an element in 1774 by the Swedish chemists Carl Scheele and Johann Ghan. It was determined to be essential for mammals in 1931 after studies showed that it was required for growth in mice and reproduction in rats.

FUNCTION

Manganese is a key component in energy metabolism. It is found in the mitochondria of cells—the powerhouses where energy is made. It is also a component of many enzymes, including the antioxidant super oxide dismutase (SOD), which participates in the body's natural anti-inflammatory reactions.

Manganese assists in synthesis of cartilage, bone, and connective tissue. It contributes to the formation of the cartilage matrix, which is found at the end of bones like a cap or shield and protects the bone from being injured by repetitive joint motion. Manganese may thus help prevent osteoarthritis.

Manganese also plays a role in the synthesis of neuro-transmitters, the chemical messengers of the brain and nervous system.

RDA AND ODI

Recommended Daily Allowance

Children, up to 11 years: 3 mg
Males and females, 11 years and older: 2 to 5 mg

Optimal Daily Intake

Males and females, 11 to 50 years: 5 mg
Males and females 50 years and older: 10 mg

DEFICIENCY SIGNS AND SYMPTOMS

True manganese deficiency is uncommon in humans. In laboratory animals, manganese deficiencies lead to skeletal defects, such as shortening and thickening of the bone, skull deformities, and joint swelling (Shils and Young, 1988). In a study of humans who were fed a manganese-deficient diet, increased calcium, phosphorus, and an enzyme called alkaline phosphatase were found. Alkaline phosphatase appears in the blood when bone demineralization has occurred. This suggests that the body utilizes the manganese present in bone to fulfill the mineral's other more pressing duties. Other symptoms noted in the study were a fine scaly rash and decreased high-density lipoprotein (HDL) cholesterol (Freeland-Graves, 1988).

Box 17.1 shows some conditions that may be treated with increased manganese intake.

BOX 17.1

CONDITIONS THAT MAY BE TREATED WITH
INCREASED MANGANESE INTAKE

Inflammatory diseases
Osteoporosis
Sprains and strains

INTERACTIONS AND FACTORS AFFECTING ABSORPTION

Iron supplementation can lead to increased manganese excretion. High intake of refined carbohydrates can lead to decreased manganese levels.

Manganese may interfere with the absorption of iron, copper, and zinc. Conversely, high doses of magnesium, calcium, iron, copper, and zinc may inhibit the absorption of manganese.

TOXICITY AND CONTRAINDICATIONS

Toxicity from dietary manganese has not been documented, but since manganese competes with iron absorption, iron-deficiency anemia is a possible contraindication.

True toxicity from manganese dust and fumes has been seen in miners, especially in Chile. The inhalation of high quantities of manganese dust results in a curious syndrome known as "manganese madness." Initially, the miners become manic with uncontrollable fits of laughter, increased libido, insomnia, delusions, and hallucinations. Later, they become severely de-

BOX 17.2
FOOD THAT CONTAIN MANGANESE
(IN LOOSE ORDER FROM HIGHEST TO LOWEST
MANGANESE CONTENT)

Whole wheat flour	Brazil nuts
Peas	Spinach
Brown rice	Almonds
Barley	Rhubarb
Rye	Beans
Buckwheat	Lettuce
Bananas	Oats
Pecans	Sweet potatoes

pressed, sleeping all the time, suffering from impotence and slow speech. This finally progresses into a condition similar to Parkinson's disease. The treatment, L-Dopa, is the same for both maladies. Evidence suggests that in huge doses manganese may interfere with the neurotransmitter dopamine.

FOOD SOURCES

Rich food sources of manganese include nuts and whole grains especially high in the germ moiety. Black tea is a good source. Meat poultry, fish, and dairy are generally poor manganese sources. See Box 17.2 for a list of foods high in manganese.

CHAPTER 18

MOLYBDENUM

Molybdenum is beginning to receive more attention these days because of its role in the detoxification of several substances, especially alcohol and sulfites.

FUNCTION

Molybdenum is essential to the function of several enzymes that are involved in the breakdown of alcohol and sulfites and in the formation of uric acid (Sardesai, 1993). Uric acid is a by-product of protein metabolism. Although uric acid has a bad reputation for causing gout, a form of arthritis, uric acid in normal amounts may be a powerful antioxidant (Hendler, 1990).

Molybdenum activates an enzyme that prevents the formation carcinogenic nitrosamines (Hendler, 1990). A deficiency of molybdenum in the soil in the Hunan Province in China, coupled with a low dietary intake of vitamin C, has been thought to be the cause of a high rate of esophageal cancer in those parts. Molybdenum supplementation is currently being undertaken in Hunan Province in an attempt to correct this situation (Luo et al., 1983).

RDA AND ODI

There is no established recommended daily allowance or optimal daily intake for molybdenum, but it is estimated that humans need 150 to 500 micrograms per day.

DEFICIENCY SIGNS AND SYMPTOMS

Molybdenum deficiency is extremely rare. There is one known case of actual deficiency in a man who was being fed intravenously. He developed a fast heart rate, increased respiration, visual disturbances, and eventually became comatose.

In animal studies, molybdenum deficiency has been linked to an increased susceptibility to sulfite toxicity and disturbances in uric acid metabolism, as well as an increased incidence of infertility and accumulation of copper in the liver and brain (Shils and Young, 1988).

One condition that may be treated with an increased intake of molybdenum is asthma. In addition, the mineral may help prevent some types of cancer.

INTERACTIONS AND FACTORS AFFECTING ABSORPTION

High doses of molybdenum may decrease copper levels in the body. It also competes with tungsten for absorption.

TOXICITY AND CONTRAINDICATIONS

Because molybdenum can increase the uric acid levels in the blood, it is not recommended for people who have problems with gout.

BOX 18.1

FOODS THAT CONTAIN MOLYBDENUM
(IN LOOSE ORDER FROM HIGHEST TO
LOWEST MOLYBDENUM CONTENT)

Lamb	Potatoes
Barley	Oats
Green beans	Cantaloupe
Lentils	Whole wheat
Squash	Corn
Strawberries	Rye bread
Carrots	Apricots
Split peas	Brewer's yeast
Green peas	Garlic
Brown rice	Molasses
Spinach	Raisins

FOOD SOURCES

The best sources of molybdenum are lamb, barley, green beans, lentils, squash, strawberries, and carrots. It is also found in the grains and in legumes. See Box 18.1 for a more complete list of foods that contain the mineral.

CHAPTER 19

PHOSPHORUS

Phosphorus and calcium have a balancing effect on each other. High levels of phosphorus cause an increased requirement for calcium in the blood. Unfortunately, when our diet is short in calcium, our systems borrow it from our bones. The average American diet is quite high in phosphorus and comparably low in calcium, due in part to our high consumption of carbonated soft drinks.

Despite the negative effect of too much phosphorus, we must be aware that it is vital to our health. It is the second most abundant mineral in our bodies and may account for close to 1.5 pounds of our total body weight (Shauss, 1995).

FUNCTIONS

Phosphorus, like calcium, is vital for strong bones and healthy teeth. It aids in the mineralization process that gives bone its density and strength.

Phosphorus is also a component of cellular membranes. The cellular membrane defines the cells boundaries, keeping the internal components inside the cell and external materials out. It also regulates the passage of material into the cell.

RDA AND ODI

The recommended daily allowance and optimal daily intake for phosphorus are identical.

Males and Females
11 to 24 years: 1,200 mg
25 years and older: 800 mg
Pregnant or lactating women: 1,200 mg

Deficiency Signs and Symptoms

Phosphorus is naturally present in many foods. It is also found in soda and food additives. Deficiency in the United States is fairly rare. People who consume large amounts of antacids, infants who are fed cow's milk, and alcoholics are most likely to develop phosphorus deficiency. People with malabsorption problems, kidney disease, and diabetic ketoacidosis are also at risk (Hendler, 1990).

The signs and symptoms of phosphorus deficiency are fatigue, weakness, and a decreased attention span. In severe cases, a phosphorus deficiency can lead to seizures, coma, and even death.

Americans eat almost four times the recommended daily allowance for phosphorus, which can lead to calcium deficiency. The body will take calcium from the bones in order to balance phosphorus levels in the blood. Thus, the development of osteoporosis may be partially linked to an overabundance of phosphorus in the diet (Hendler, 1990).

There are no known conditions that may be treated with an increased intake in phosphorus.

INTERACTIONS AND FACTORS AFFECTING ABSORPTION

Phosphorus absorption, like calcium, is enhanced in an acidic environment. Iron, magnesium, and aluminum all decrease its

> ## BOX 19.1
> ## FOODS THAT CONTAIN PHOSPHORUS
>
> Meat
> Poultry
> Fish
> Eggs
> Cheese

absorption. Antacids containing aluminum and magnesium bind to phosphorus and make it impossible for the body to absorb.

Phosphorus and calcium must be maintained at about a 1:1 ratio in the diet. An excess of either will cause the other to be extracted from the bones and tissues.

TOXICITY AND CONTRAINDICATIONS

Too much phosphorus in the system can inhibit calcium absorption and lead to problems such as osteoporosis or other related conditions associated with calcium deficiency. Excess phosphorus can also cause diarrhea.

FOOD SOURCES

The best source of phosphorus is from animal foods. See Box 19.1 for a more complete list.

CHAPTER 20

SELENIUM

Named for Selene, the Roman goddess of the moon, selenium was discovered in 1817 by the Swedish scientist Jons Jacob Berzelius. This mineral is unevenly distributed in the earth's crust, with some areas, such as large parts of the Great Plains and Southern California, containing high quantities in the soil. The soils of other areas, such as the Eastern Seaboard and Pacific Northwest, have low selenium content.

Earlier in this century selenium was known only as a toxic mineral. Livestock animals in the American West develop selenium toxicity when they eat large amounts of "locoweed," a name for some plants of the *astragalus* genus. The condition, known as alkali disease, causes problems such as hair loss, liver cirrhosis, lameness, and hoof malformations.

Insufficient selenium can also cause problems for animals. Livestock that lack it in their diets eventually develop deficiency diseases. It was not until 1957 that scientists realized that selenium is essential not just for animals, but for humans as well.

FUNCTION

Selenium's function can be summed up in one concept: protection. Selenium is a key component of the enzyme glutathione peroxidase, which protects the body from a vast array of harmful substances by breaking down toxins, protecting cells from damage by free radicals, and binding heavy metals such as cadmium and mercury.

As an antioxidant and detoxifier of toxic substances selenium appears to protect the system against damage that leads to heart disease and stroke. It strengthens immunity, enhances longevity, and detoxifies environmental pollutants (Murray, 1995). Selenium appears to work synergistically with vitamin E to prevent heart disease (Stone, 1986). These two nutrients may also help the elderly improve their mental alertness and emotional well being, decreasing depression, poor appetite, and fatigue (Schauss, 1995).

Recent research also shows that selenium plays a role in the conversion of the thyroid hormone, T_4, into the metabolically active form, T_3. Therefore, selenium deficiency may be partially implicated in some types of hypothyroidism (Contempre et al., 1992).

RDA AND ODI

Recommended Daily Allowance

Males
11 to 14 years: 40 mcg
15 to 18 years: 50 mcg
19 years and older: 70 mcg

Females
11 to 14 years: 45 mcg
15 to 18 years: 50 mcg
19 years and older: 55 mcg

Optimal Daily Intake

Males

11 to 14 years: 60 mcg
15 to 18 years: 70 mcg
19 to 24 years: 100 mcg
25 to 50 years: 175 mcg
51 years and older: 250 mcg

Females

11 to 14 years: 165 mcg
15 to 18 years: 70 mcg
19 to 24 years: 90 mcg
25 to 50 years: 175 mcg
51 years and older: 200 mcg

DEFICIENCY SIGNS AND SYMPTOMS

Selenium deficiency is a growing problem. This may be due in part to the leaching of the soil by modern agricultural methods. But environmental pollution may also play a role in the depletion of selenium. There is a possibility that sulfur dioxide fallout and acid rain may compete with selenium for uptake into plants, thereby decreasing their selenium content (Hendler, 1990).

Areas with decreased amounts of selenium in the soil have an increased incidence of heart disease. In certain areas of China, many people suffer from a disease of the heart muscle called Keshan disease. Fatal in nearly 50 percent of those who suffer from it, Keshan disease continued to recur in dispersed areas year after year, baffling doctors and scientists. Eventually they discovered that the common factor in these areas was selenium-deficient soil. In 1974, a large-scale study gave selenium supplements to more than eleven thousand children and

---

BOX 20.1
THERAPEUTIC USES FOR SELENIUM

Arthritis	Cataract prevention
Atherosclerosis prevention	Muscular dystrophy
Cancer prevention	prevention
Heart attack prevention	Male infertility
Immunodeficiency	Heavy metal toxicity

---

placebos to nine thousand children. Those who received only placebos developed 106 cases of Keshan disease; fifty-three of them died. But those who received selenium developed only nineteen cases of Keshan disease and suffered only one death. Since then, selenium has been regularly supplemented in China, and the disease has virtually disappeared.

Selenium deficiency can also result in infertility, sudden infant death syndrome, cystic fibrosis, chronic fatigue syndrome, muscular dystrophy, liver cirrhosis, and many other conditions (Wallach and Lan, 1994).

Box 20.1 shows some therapeutic uses for selenium.

INTERACTIONS AND FACTORS AFFECTING ABSORPTION

Inorganic forms of selenium, such as sodium selenate or sodium selenite, are poorly absorbed, especially when combined with vitamin C. There is also evidence that these forms have an increased likelihood of toxicity.

L-selenomethionine is the form of selenium that is found in food and is also the most readily absorbed. Other antioxidants,

---

BOX 20.2
FOODS THAT CONTAIN SELENIUM

Brazil nuts	Wheat germ
Snapper	Blackstrap molasses
Halibut	Sunflower seeds
Salmon	Granola
Scallops	Whole wheat bread
Swiss chard	Brown rice
Clams	Turnips
Oats	Barley, raw
Orange juice	Garlic
Oysters	

---

particularly vitamin E, act synergistically with selenium to increase the activity of glutathione peroxidase. Heavy metals decrease the absorption of selenium.

TOXICITY AND CONTRAINDICATIONS

Selenium is toxic in minute doses, with a very narrow margin of safety. It is generally recommended to keep any supplementation between 50 and 200 *micrograms*. Higher doses than this, taken over a period of time, have been associated with toxicity.

Signs of selenium toxicity include nausea and vomiting, emotional instability, a garlic odor on the breath and skin, and, in extreme cases, loss of hair and fingernails. Long-term high dosages of selenium have been linked to liver, skeletal, and cardiac damage. High levels of selenium have also been found to be carcinogenic.

Selenium appears to lose some of its beneficial functions when exposed to lead, mercury, cadmium, and arsenic. Chronic exposure to environmental toxins, including chemotherapeutic drugs and other toxic medications, increases the requirement for selenium because it is used to generate glutathione peroxidase, the enzyme that detoxifies these substances.

FOOD SOURCES

The amount of selenium present in plant food depends on the selenium levels in the soil where the food was grown. Seafood is high in selenium. See Box 20.2 for a list of good sources of the mineral.

CHAPTER 21

SILICON

Silicon dioxide is a crystalline compound found abundantly in sand, quartz, agates, flint, and many other naturally occurring materials. It was first found in the ash of animal tissue in 1848 and was added to the list of essential trace minerals in 1972. It is a part of the body structure of lower classes of species, such as sponges, algae, and certain marine protozoa. Since the turn of the century, silicon (also known as silica) has been found in high concentrations in the tendons and eye tissue of humans. It has a chemical structure similar to carbon.

FUNCTION

Silicon is important in the formation of the collagen found in bone, cartilage, and other connective tissue. The calcification sites of growing bone contain high concentrations of silicon and scientists think it contributes to the organic matrix that allows the proper mineralization of both bones and teeth (Marz, 1997).

Silicon is also necessary for the formation of other connective tissues like elastin, which help maintain the integrity of the elastic quality of blood vessels and other tissue. The highest concentrations of silicon are found in the hair and skin.

RDA AND ODI

No official recommended daily allowance has been established for silicon. An optimal daily intake is between 20 and 50 milligrams per day for adults (Marz, 1997).

DEFICIENCY SIGNS AND SYMPTOMS

Silicon deficiency has not been identified in humans. However, dry, brittle nails and hair, along with poor skin quality, may indicate a deficiency (Wallach and Lan, 1994). Induced silicon deficiency in chicks resulted in skeletal abnormalities and poor calcification of bone.

Box 21.1 shows some possible therapeutic uses for silicon.

INTERACTIONS AND FACTORS AFFECTING ABSORPTION

Fiber, molybdenum, magnesium, and fluoride elevate the silicon requirement. High-fiber diets also contain higher amounts of silicon than low-fiber diets, perhaps canceling out any negative effect of fiber (Shils and Young, 1988).

BOX 21.1

POSSIBLE THERAPEUTIC USES FOR SILICON

Aging skin, hair, fingernails
Atherosclerosis
Osteoporosis

BOX 21.2

FOODS THAT CONTAIN SILICON

Oats	Whole wheat
Beets	Turnips
Barley	White rice
Soybeans	Raisins
Brown rice	Green beans

TOXICITY AND CONTRAINDICATIONS

Dietary silicon is considered nontoxic. However, increased levels of silicon along with aluminum have been found in the brains of people with Alzheimer's disease.

There have also been some reports that long-term use of the silicon-containing antacid magnesium trisilicate has been associated with the formation of kidney stones in some people. Certain animals that eat large quantities of plants with high silicon content may also develop kidney stones.

FOOD SOURCES

Silicon is generally found in high-fiber foods, especially in the husks of grains. Keep in mind that food processing removes almost all silicon. Meats, fish, and dairy products are poor sources of silicon. See Box 21.2 for a list of the best sources of silicon.

CHAPTER 22

SULFUR

Sulfur is found throughout the human body and is included in the structure of proteins. It is an important component of many enzymes, hormones, and antibodies. Sulfur is reputed to give hair its luster and the complexion its glow. Two of the B vitamins, biotin and thiamine, contain sulfur (Murray, 1995).

FUNCTION

Sulfur is especially abundant in the skin, hair, and nails, but its functions throughout the body are varied and many. As part of the genetic material of cells, it is vital to the production of energy. It also promotes enzymatic reactions and aids in blood clotting (MacDonald, 1996). Sulfur combines with some toxic materials to allow them to pass out of the body through the urine. It is part of the antioxidant enzyme glutathione peroxidase. In addition, it is essential to the manufacture of protein, as the amino acids taurine, cystine, methionine, glutathione, and homocystine all contain the mineral. Finally, the mineral aids in bile secretion from the liver (Griffith, 1988).

Box 22.1
Foods High in Sulfur

Broccoli	Eggs
Beans	Fish
Beef (lean)	Milk
Cabbage	Whole wheat
Clams	

RDA and ODI

There is no established recommended daily allowance or optimal daily intake for sulfur.

Deficiency Signs and Symptoms

Although most experts contend that there is no such thing as sulfur deficiency, Joel Wallach, D.V.M., N.D., and M. Lan, M.D., M.S., authors of *Rare Earths: Forbidden Cures*, say a deficiency of sulfur may lead to degenerative forms of arthritis that affect the cartilage, ligaments, and tendons (Wallach and Lan, 1994). This may account for the traditional practice of soaking in sulphurous hot springs to treat arthritis pain.

There are no established conditions that may be treated by increased intake of sulfur.

Interactions and Factors Affecting Absorption

Smoking tobacco decreases the absorption of sulfur (Griffith, 1988).

TOXICITY AND CONTRAINDICATIONS

There are no known contraindications or toxicities from dietary sulfur.

FOOD SOURCES

Some animal foods and cruciferous vegetables are rich sources of sulfur. See Box 22.1 for a more complete list.

CHAPTER 23

VANADIUM

Vanadium, named after the Scandinavian goddess of beauty, youth, and luster, was used in the last century by French physicians as a treatment for diabetes and fatigue. Its popularity spread to North America, where it was used for hardening of the arteries. Once insulin was discovered, however, the use of vanadium dwindled because it can also be quite toxic (Hendler, 1990, and Shils and Young, 1988).

Vanadium was declared an essential nutrient in 1971. But the scientific information on vanadium is mixed: Although one resource calls it essential, another criticizes the studies that determined the ill effects of vanadium deficiency. The best evidence in favor of vanadium as an essential element comes from a long-term study of vanadium-deprived goats. Their offspring had bone deformities in their front legs, and some of them died within three days after birth. In addition, the vanadium-deficient mother goats produced less milk (Harland, 1994).

FUNCTION

Vanadium is involved in glucose, cholesterol, and bone metabolism. It may act independently from insulin in lowering glucose levels. It has also been found to suppress cholesterol synthesis in the livers of young people who have higher cholesterol levels. Trials in adults with higher cholesterol failed to reduce levels.

Vanadium stimulates glucose uptake into the fat cells and the transformation into glycogen for storage. In studies on diabetic rats, vanadium appears to work like insulin by stabilizing blood glucose levels in the normal range (Wallach and Lan, 1994). Vanadium also appears to make the cell membranes more sensitive to insulin.

Vanadium initiates an increase in the contractile force of the heart. Several studies indicate that it may have anticancer properties in the mammary glands of mice (McNeill, 1993, and Neilsen, 1987). Vanadium also appears to be involved in the mineralization of bone and teeth.

RDA AND OPTIMAL VALUES

No recommended daily allowance for vanadium has been established. The estimated safe and effective daily dietary intake is 100 micrograms per day, which is easily achieved in the diet.

DEFICIENCY SIGNS AND SYMPTOMS

No sign of vanadium deficiency has been consistently induced in any animal (Shils and Young, 1988). Increased intake has been used to treat diabetes, as the mineral lowers blood glucose levels.

INTERACTIONS AND FACTORS
AFFECTING ABSORPTION

Increased levels of vanadium have been found in hair samples of patients with bipolar disorder. Lithium, the drug of choice for the treatment of manic depression, may work by reversing

---

BOX 23.1

FOODS THAT CONTAIN VANADIUM

(IN LOOSE ORDER FROM HIGHEST TO

LOWEST VANADIUM CONTENT)

Dill seeds	Tomatoes
Black pepper	Parsley
Mushrooms	Carrots
Shellfish	Olive oil
Buckwheat groats	Whole wheat
Corn	Sunflower seeds
Oats	Apples
Green beans	Beets

---

some of the ill effects of these high levels of vanadium (Harland and Harden-Williams, 1993).

TOXICITY AND CONTRAINDICATIONS

Dosages higher than 250 micrograms per day of vanadium may be very dangerous. Symptoms of toxicity in animals include suppression of the immune system, destruction of red blood cells, and even death (Schauss, 1995). This may be due to the type of vanadium used, however. Vandate appears to be considerably more toxic than vanadyl sulfate.

Human studies have not yet produced the same serious side effects. However, high doses over a long period of time have produced diarrhea and abdominal cramps (Murray, 1996). In addition, high doses of vanadium may deplete vitamin C (Harland and Harden-Williams, 1994).

FOOD SOURCES

Vanadium appears only in small quantities in food. The richest sources are certain spices, such as dill seeds, parsley, and black pepper. Mushrooms, shellfish, and grains also contain fairly high levels. Lower quantities are found in meat, fish, and poultry. Some good sources of dietary vanadium are listed in Box 23.1.

CHAPTER 24

ZINC

Dwarfism was once common in the mountainous villages of Iran, affecting up to 3 percent of the male population. The usual diet in these villages consisted of unleavened bread with small amounts of milk and potatoes. Fruits, vegetables, meats, and eggs were very seldom consumed. Men who suffered from this condition, characterized by severe anemia, underdeveloped genitals, and poor physical development, responded rapidly to zinc supplementation in their diets. Thus zinc, which had been recognized as an essential trace mineral in animals since 1934, was finally accepted as essential for humans in 1972 (Shils and Young, 1988).

The men who suffered from dwarfism consumed diets high in zinc, but the unleavened grains they ate also contained high quantities of phytic acid, which binds to zinc, creating an insoluble compound that the body can't absorb. The dietary addition of meat, seafood, seeds, beans, and cheeses provide zinc in a form that can easily be absorbed.

Zinc is found in virtually every cell in the body and is a component in more than two hundred enzymes. It is stored in the muscle and concentrated in the white and red blood cells. High levels of zinc are normally found in men's prostate glands. Fingernails and toenails, hair, eyes, liver, and skin also contain zinc.

FUNCTION

Zinc is essential to cell growth and replication, sexual maturation, fertility and reproduction, night vision, immune defenses, taste, and appetite. The most significant consequence of a zinc deficiency is impaired growth (Shils and Young, 1988).

Zinc helps in the transfer of carbon dioxide—the waste product of cellular energy production—from the cells to the lungs for exhalation. It is also important in the calcification of bones and for the development and proper functioning of the reproductive organs. Zinc plays a vital role in several enzyme systems that are involved in digestion and respiration. Insulin, which regulates blood sugar, needs zinc to function properly.

Zinc works with vitamin A in vision, human reproduction, and cell reproduction. Without proper levels of zinc, people have trouble adjusting their eyes to see in the dark. A deficiency of zinc can also result in any number of skin disorders, and it is important in healing burns and wounds.

Zinc promotes immune system functions in a variety of ways. The thymus gland, the master gland of the immune system, requires zinc to make its hormones. Natural killer cells—specialized immune cells that kill tumor cells and virally infected cells—also need zinc to function properly. Our brain and central nervous system require zinc for almost every enzymatic reaction.

RDA AND ODI

Recommended Daily Allowance

Males, 11 years and older: 15 mg
Females, 11 years and older: 12 mg
Females, pregnant and lactating: 20 mg
Infants: 5 mg

Optimal Daily Intake

Males
11 to 14 years: 15 mg
15 to 18 years: 18 mg
19 years and older: 20 mg

Females
11 to 14 years: 12 mg
15 to 18 years: 15 mg
19 years and older: 17 mg

DEFICIENCY SIGNS AND SYMPTOMS

Zinc deficiencies are most commonly caused by low zinc in the diet, excess reliance on grains, and heavy alcohol use. Women who are pregnant or breastfeeding are more susceptible to zinc deficiencies. The elderly are also particularly vulnerable, primarily because of low dietary zinc content and lowered capacity for absorption.

Zinc requirements increase during times of healing and recovery. Children with allergies also need more zinc than usual. Other people who commonly suffer from zinc deficiencies are those with conditions such as diabetes, chronic liver disease, kidney disease, sickle cell anemia, malabsorption, and premenstrual syndrome. People who are on estrogen, corticosteroids, antiseizure medication, or diuretics are also susceptible to zinc deficiencies.

Pica, a condition where children and sometimes adult women develop cravings for indigestible items, such as laundry starch, dirt, and lead paint, may be associated with a zinc deficiency, especially in children ages one to three. Pica is also associated with iron and calcium deficiencies (Marz, 1997).

Zinc deficiency is characterized by loss of appetite, stunted growth in children, small sex glands in boys, loss of taste sensitivity, and dull hair. Many different skin disorders, including eczema, acne, and psoriasis, are related to zinc deficiency. Other problems associated with low zinc levels are infertility, mouth ulcers, growth retardation, and sleep disorders. Some people associate white spots on the fingernails with zinc deficiency. This is thought to reflect poor wound healing, which is also associated with zinc deficiency, since white spots are probably due to trauma to the nail bed (Murray, 1996). Zinc deficiency can result in decreased numbers of antibodies and lymphocytes, leading to increased susceptibility to infection.

The prostate gland needs zinc to protect it from the action of an enzyme known as 5-alpha reductase, which converts testosterone into dihydrotestosterone. Zinc deficiency leads to the accumulation of dihydrotestosterone in the prostate, causing the gland to swell, in turn affecting the urinary flow in many older men — a condition known as benign prostatic hyperplasia or BPH.

Some psychiatric illnesses, all types of inflammatory bowel disease, impaired glucose tolerance, arthritis, alcoholism, and dandruff have all been correlated to zinc deficiency. Decreased senses of taste and smell may also be related to low zinc levels.

Box 24.1 shows some conditions that may be treated with increased zinc intake.

INTERACTIONS AND FACTORS AFFECTING ABSORPTION

Vitamin A is necessary for the absorption and metabolism of zinc. Zinc absorption is enhanced by soy protein, red wine, glucose, and lactose. Vitamin B_6 may also enhance its absorption.

Zinc absorption is inhibited by copper, iron, manganese, and high calcium. Cadmium replaces zinc in the body. Phytates, which are often found in foods that contain zinc, such as nuts,

BOX 24.1
CONDITIONS THAT MAY BE TREATED
WITH INCREASED ZINC INTAKE

Acne	Immunodepression
AIDS/HIV	Infertility (in males)
Anorexia nervosa	Intestinal ulcers and
Benign prostatic	infections
hyperplasia	Macular degeneration
Cataracts	Psoriasis
Eczema	Poor wound healing
Herpes infections	Rheumatoid arthritis

seeds, whole grains, and legumes, bond to zinc, making it impossible for the body to absorb. Diuretics decrease zinc absorption by increasing excretion. Oral contraceptives lower blood levels of zinc. Zinc decreases the amount of tetracycline absorbed in the blood, thereby decreasing its efficiency. Zinc and tetracycline should be taken at least two hours apart.

Of the forms of zinc supplements, zinc sulfate appears to be the most easily absorbed. However, zinc chelates—acetate, citrate, glycerate, picolinate—are all absorbed well, too.

TOXICITY AND CONTRAINDICATIONS

High doses of zinc can cause nausea and stomach upset. Zinc supplementation over a long period of time can cause a copper deficiency because it competes with copper for absorption. Zinc should always be taken with copper in a 10:1 to 30:1 zinc-to-copper ratio.

Zinc supplementation may lower high-density lipoprotein (HDL) cholesterol, which is the good type of cholesterol, and raise cholesterol levels in general. Too much zinc may also impair immunity, cause skin rashes and depression, and reduce tolerance of alcohol. Large doses of zinc may also promote folate deficiency (Marz, 1997).

FOOD SOURCES

Oysters are the best known and highest quantity source of zinc. Shellfish, red meat, and fish all contain high zinc concentrations as well. See Box 24.2 for the best sources of zinc.

Zinc is also found in nuts, seeds, whole grains, and legumes, but the phytic acid content in these foods may make the zinc unavailable for absorption by the body. Food processing removes a good portion of zinc as well as other trace elements. For example, whole brown rice has more than four times the zinc that polished white rice has. Molasses has forty-two times more zinc than an equal amount of white sugar. Per weight, the germ part of wheat has fifteen times more zinc than white flour.

BOX 24.2
THE BEST SOURCES OF ZINC

Oysters	Swiss cheese
Ginger root	Swiss chard
Beef	Sesame tahini
Peas, dried	Crab
Turkey, dark meat	Mustard greens
Leek	Fermented soy products
Cheddar cheese	Tuna

CHAPTER 25

Minerals and Disease

In Chapters 5 through 24 I described the essential minerals in detail, explained their role in human physiology, and named some symptoms and conditions that their deficiency may cause or contribute to. In this chapter, I'll show the progression of the pathology of mineral deficiency *as a group* rather than singly. I'll also list groups of mineral deficiencies associated with some specific illnesses.

The Conventional Model of a Deficiency Disease

The conventional scientific approach to mineral-deficiency diseases is modeled on the germ theory of disease: A single germ causes a single disease. In other words, medical scientists require proof that the deficiency of a single mineral causes a single deficiency disease (see the introduction to Section 2). That model, however, does not fit the reality of human diet and nutrition, especially in the case of minerals. Mineral elements do not exist alone in foods. In natural foods, they come as a group that includes the essential minerals and dozens of other trace elements. Minerals in a natural diet of animal and plant foods are also accompanied by vitamins, essential fatty acids and other beneficial fats, fiber, and dozens of other beneficial constituents. We saw in Chapters 5 to 24 that these constituents, especially the minerals, vitamins, fiber, and fatty acids, have complex interactions. Trying to isolate the effect of a single nutrient is like trying to take one color from the rainbow. When we develop deficiencies, we develop them as a group. Most of the Western diseases are associated with *multiple* deficiencies, not deficiencies of a single nutrient (see Table 2.8.).

Conventional medicine often does not recognize the early stages and symptoms of a mineral or vitamin deficiency. Scientists wait until a fully developed organic disease occurs, such as anemia, osteoporosis, or goiter. The normal pathology of a mineral deficiency disease is:

1. Deficient intake in the diet.
2. Levels drop in the blood and extracellular fluid.
3. The body robs the bones and tissues to maintain steady levels in the fluids.
4. Deficiencies in the tissues result first in the form of *functional diseases* because the cells cannot perform their roles at an optimal level.
5. Eventually, the tissues themselves become deformed or deranged, and *organic disease* results.

For example, a calcium deficiency in the diet causes a loss of calcium in the bones, nerves, and other tissues, while blood levels remain steady. The first symptoms may be depression, insomnia, anxiety, and muscle cramps. A recent scientific trial found that a group of depressed women had bone density 10 percent lower than a nondepressed group. The first-stage functional disease—depression—was present, but the bones had not yet deteriorated enough to diagnose osteoporosis (Michelson et

al., 1996). Eventually, high blood pressure may develop, and finally, osteoporosis. Of those conditions, medical scientists iden-
tify only osteoporosis as a calcium-deficiency disease, although
some kinds of high blood pressure are an organic disease of the
arteries.

In a similar process, when a magnesium deficiency occurs
in the diet, the body robs the tissues of stored magnesium. Muscle weakness, fatigue, nervousness, and irritability are the first
functional diseases to appear. Eventually, as the body loots the
magnesium stores in the heart muscle out of necessity, the
heart's function becomes impaired. Ultimately, the magnesium
deficiency causes an excess of calcium in the blood and kidney
stones—and an organic rather than functional disease may appear. Although some scientific studies show the correlation between magnesium deficiency and anxiety, muscle weakness,
fatigue, and functional heart disease, the conventional scientific
bodies do not label these as deficiency diseases. Magnesium
deficiency is not the *only* thing that causes or contributes to
these conditions, so they do not fit the definition of a deficiency
disease.

This strict standard for proving a deficiency disease—that
a single nutrient must cause a single organic deficiency disease—is partly responsible for the medical establishment's
shocking lack of insight into the contribution of mineral deficiencies to our most common and deadly illnesses.

THE PATHOLOGY OF MULTIPLE MINERAL DEFICIENCIES

Trowell and Burkitt described the progression of pathology of
organic Western diseases (see Chapter 2). Obesity, an organic
disease, appears first, followed by diabetes. Hypertension, an
organic disease of the arteries, appears first, followed by stroke,

kidney damage, and finally heart attack. The full pathology of Western deficiency diseases should include the functional diseases that appear first. In the sections that follow, I will present my view of this pathological progression. You will see that deficiency diseases do not progress the way they would in a laboratory, but are complicated by the side effects of addictive substances in foods, prescription and non-prescription drugs, and surgery.

The Deficient Diet

In Chapter 2, I described the most important dietary changes that apparently cause or contribute to the development of the Western diseases. They are the introduction of sugar, refined flour, canned foods, and meat that is deficient in essential fatty acids. Box 25.1 shows the top ten sources of calories in the American diet. It should be clear from the discussion in Chapter 2 that these caloric sources are at the root of many of

---

Box 25.1

Top Ten Sources of Calories in the American Diet

1. Whole milk
2. Cola
3. Margarine
4. White bread
5. Rolls, ready to serve
6. Sugar
7. Milk (2% milk fat)
8. Ground beef
9. Wheat flour (white)
10. Pasteurized processed American cheese

the Western diseases today. I will discuss milk, margarine, and cheese in Chapter 26.

Stage 1: Functional Diseases

The first effects of broad-spectrum deficiency diseases are usually felt in the emotional life and energy level. Depression, anxiety, insomnia, mental imbalance, and fatigue are all associated with multiple deficiencies (see Table 25.1). The source for the information in Table 25.1 is *Nutritional Influences on Mental Illness* by Dr. Melvyn Werbach, a compilation of summaries of

TABLE 25.1 NUTRIENTS ASSOCIATED
WITH FUNCTIONAL
DEFICIENCY DISEASES

Condition	Minerals	Vitamins	Other
Aggressive behavior	iron lithium	thiamine vitamin C	high sugar high cow's milk
Allergies	calcium magnesium zinc	niacin pantothenic acid vitamin B_{12} vitamin C vitamin E	essential fatty acids
Anxiety	calcium magnesium	pyridoxine niacin thiamine	high calcium high sugar high caffeine high alcohol essential fatty acids

(continues)

TABLE 25.1 *(continued)*

Condition	Minerals	Vitamins	Other
Depression	calcium copper iron lithium magnesium potassium rubidium	biotin folic acid pyridoxine riboflavin thiamine vitamin B_{12} vitamin C	high caffeine high sugar
Fatigue	iron magnesium potassium zinc	folic acid pantothenic acid pyridoxine vitamin B_{12} vitamin C vitamin E	high sugar high caffeine
Hyperactivity	calcium copper iron magnesium zinc high aluminum high lead	niacin pyridoxine thiamine	high sugar
Immunodepression	copper germanium iodine iron magnesium manganese selenium zinc	vitamin A folic acid pantothenic acid riboflavin vitamin B_6 vitamin B_{12} vitamin C vitamin D vitamin E	high sugar
Insomnia	copper iron magnesium high aluminum		high caffeine high alcohol

scientific studies. While scientific consensus may not exist for the associations with each of the nutrient deficiencies in the table, at least one peer-reviewed scientific article has appeared for each. I've also included the nutrient deficiencies associated with immunodepression and allergies, first-stage functional diseases characterized by frequent colds, flu, and heightened allergic responses. This information comes from Werbach's other book of scientific abstracts, *Nutritional Influences on Illness* (1993). Review the tables in Chapter 2 that show the nutrient losses that accompany a diet of modern foods, and you will find many of the same nutrients associated with these functional illnesses. Table 4.3 also includes functional symptoms associated with deficiencies of some of the minerals.

Stage 2: Self-Medication with Food and Drugs

With the onset of these conditions, individuals usually self-medicate with stimulants, sedatives, and/or recreational drugs. Box 25.2 shows the top ten items sold in U.S. grocery stores in 1990. Seven of the ten items contain drugs: nicotine, caffeine, or alcohol. Three contain sugar, which Box 25.1 also ranks as the sixth leading source of calories for Americans. Sugar is an "energy drug," giving a brief burst of energy and mental stimulation. The mental and emotional discomfort of nutrient deficiencies can also drive some individuals to use recreational drugs such as marijuana. In addition, people consume over-the-counter stimulants, sedatives, and pain and cold medications by the hundreds of tons annually. Per capita expenditures on nonprescription drugs in the United States rose from about $120 a year in 1986 to more than $160 in 1995 (figures adjusted for inflation in 1982 dollars), for total annual sales approaching $40 billion (U.S. Department of Commerce, 1989, 1996).

Nutrient deficiencies underlie or contribute to many addictions. Improvement of the diet can assist greatly in recovery, presumably by removing mental and emotional functional diseases that accompany the addiction. In a clinical trial in an alcohol recovery center, two groups of chronic alcoholics were given the identical therapy, except that one group received nutrition education. Classes included basic nutrition and how to shop and prepare healthy foods. At the end of a year, more than 70 percent of the group that received nutrition education were still in recovery, while about 80 percent of the control group had left recovery and returned to drinking (Beasley, 1992).

Stage 3: Prescription Drugs for Functional Diseases

Eventually, self-medication with over-the-counter drugs fails to resolve the symptoms and discomfort of functional diseases. In this stage, prescription drugs—such as antibiotics, antidepressants, and sedatives—replace or supplement the substances already in use. Side effects of prescription drugs exacerbate the existing deficiencies. In 1984, the per capita annual

---

BOX 25.2

TOP TEN ITEMS SOLD IN U.S.
GROCERY STORES (1990)

1. Marlboro cigarettes
2. Coca-Cola Classic
3. Pepsi-Cola
4. Kraft American cheese
5. Diet Coke
6. Campbell's soup
7. Budweiser beer
8. Tide detergent
9. Folger's coffee
10. Winston cigarettes

CASE STUDY #1

A fifty-year-old man complained of mental confusion and memory loss on intake at my clinic. The mental confusion caused him to frequently lose study items necessary for a course of higher education he was pursuing, and he had been fired from a job. A review of his diet showed a typical Western diet containing almost no nutritious foods in their natural state. He revealed that his underlying problem was insomnia, from which he had suffered for more than ten years. For nine of those years, he had taken an over-the-counter sleep medication *every night* to go to sleep. His severe mental confusion was a side effect of the drug.

CASE STUDY #2

A forty-two-year-old woman initially complained of blurred vision and ringing in the ears. During the interview, she revealed that she also suffered from severe heartburn, and that a sprained knee was healing very slowly. The blurred vision, ringing in the ears, and heartburn were side effects of an over-the-counter pain medication she was taking regularly for her sprained knee. Her diet was typically American, and the resulting deficiencies, as well as the drug side effects, were probably contributing to the slow healing of her knee (anti-inflammatory medications that suppress pain also suppress healing).

expenditure in the United States for prescription drugs was $1,200. By 1995, the figure reached $2,820 in 1984 dollars— more than double—or $4,117 in real dollars (U.S. Department of Commerce, 1996). Much of this is paid for by health insurance, Medicare, and other third-party payers.

Stage 4: Onset of Chronic Organic Disease

Because the initial nutrient deficiencies have not been addressed, the diseases progress to the organic stage. The first to appear is usually obesity. Since 1980, the percentage of the population classified as obese has increased from 25 percent to 33 percent. Other common early stage organic diseases caused by the Western diet are arthritis, atherosclerosis, autoimmune diseases, hypertension, skin conditions, and ulcerative diseases. See Table 2.5 for some of the nutrients associated with these conditions. In addition to the conditions listed there, peptic ulcers have been associated with deficiencies of calcium, magnesium, and zinc — three of the most common deficiencies in our society. At this stage, even more prescription drugs are consumed, on a permanent basis, with more side effects. A good number of Americans over sixty are at this stage of pathology (see Table 25.2 and Box 25.3). You might suppose that the prescription drugs older Americans take are necessary to maintain their health. For an alternative opinion, based on medical expert testimony and advice, see the book *Worst Pills, Best Pills II* by Dr. Sidney Wolfe and pharmacist Rose-Ellen Hope (1993). The authors conclude that about two-thirds of these drugs are either unnecessary or inappropriately prescribed. Because I'm including data on older Americans here, do not think that we experience chronic organic disease only in our elder years. Many children suffer from obesity and other early stage organic diseases before they are old enough to enter school.

Stage 5: Life-Threatening or Fatal Organic Disease

The leading causes of death in our society come from the end stages of organic Western diseases — heart disease, cancer, and stroke. See Tables 2.8, 4.3, and 4.4 for some nutrients associated with these diseases. At this stage, poor health is made

CASE STUDY #3

A forty-six-year-old woman complained of depression and loss of sex drive. She was a vegetarian and ate many modern foods, including sugar and white flour. The resulting deficiencies contributed to her depression. A prescription antidepressant drug was causing the loss of libido, which did not appear until a few months after she started taking the drug.

CASE STUDY #4

A twenty-two-year-old woman had suffered from attacks of systemic lupus for two years. Her current diet contained some nutritious foods, but also included fast foods such as pizza. The beneficial foods in the diet had been a recent addition. A review of her complete medical history showed steroid prescriptions for fungal infections and eczema as an infant, frequent antibiotic prescriptions for upper respiratory infections as a young child, and multiple antibiotic and antifungal prescriptions later in childhood and teenage years for urinary tract infections. A review of her diet suggested a lifelong allergy to dairy products, and her most serious lupus symptoms stopped with removal of that food. She also had pain and discomfort in every level of the digestive tract. The repeated antibiotic medications had damaged the lining of her gut, allowing bowel bacteria and foods to flow into the system, initiating or exacerbating the complex immune reactions of the lupus.

TABLE 25.2   PRESCRIPTION DRUGS IN OLDER
AMERICANS (60 AND OLDER)*

Treatment Type	Percentage of Older Americans
Taking five or more prescriptions	37
Taking seven or more prescriptions	19
Taking a cardiovascular drug	65
Taking an antidepressant or sedative	33
Taking a gastrointestinal drug (for constipation, ulcers, colitis)	24

(Source: Wolfe and Hope, 1993)

* Average prescriptions filled per year is 15.4. Data does not include elders in nursing homes

---

BOX 25.3

THE MOST COMMON SIDE EFFECTS
OF PRESCRIPTION DRUGS

Drugs often complicate the symptoms of simple deficiency diseases. Here are the most common side effects to prescription drugs.

Constipation
Depression
Sexual dysfunction
Memory loss
Hallucinations
Insomnia
Parkinsonism

(Source: Wolfe and Hope, 1993)

CASE STUDY #5

A seventy-two-year-old woman had simultaneous diagnoses of psoriasis, psoriatic arthritis, rheumatoid arthritis, ulcerative colitis, liver cancer, and lung cancer. She was on more than seven drug prescriptions, including two chemotherapy agents. She had been prescribed a powerful drug—methotrexate—for the psoriasis and arthritis and had taken it for more than seven years. Her ailments were Western diseases, presumably with nutritional components. According to her own doctors, the methotrexate had caused the liver and lung cancers. According to standard pharmaceutical references, the drug can also cause ulcerative diseases of the intestines, which, in her case, appeared only after taking the drug.

---

worse by more drugs, surgical procedures, and even organ removal.

CONCLUSION

We saw in Chapter 2 that most of the conditions discussed in this chapter can be attributed to the Western diet. They do not appear in primitive people consuming a traditional diet of whole foods and wild game, but begin to appear when those people begin to consume Western foods. It is true that genetics, environmental factors, and other things beyond our control also contribute to these conditions. Yet the results of anthropological studies point to diet as the primary cause. In the next section, I will discuss dietary changes that may improve these conditions. In the case of chronic organic diseases complicated by drug side effects, it may be too late for a complete cure.

However, most people at *any* stage start to feel much better when they switch to a natural whole-foods diet. The "cure" usually progresses in the same order as the disease pathology, with functional illnesses such as depression, anxiety, insomnia, and fatigue clearing up first. You may feel better, happier, sleep better, have more energy, suffer fewer infections and allergic symptoms, and so on. In most of the cases I've seen, people who begin to eat this way with dedication begin to feel much better within about ten days.

GETTING THE MINERALS YOU NEED

IN THIS section I will describe some mineral-rich foods available today, criticize some of the fad diets in vogue now—including the lowfat diet—and tell you how to shop for and use supplements. The recommendations I make in this section are based first of all on my own clinical experience within the tradition of nature cure. Over the last twenty-five years, I have also personally modified my diet a number of times, including trials with various fad diets. I currently practice what I preach in this section.

My experience, both personally and in a practitioner/ client setting, did not come out of thin air. I constantly read the literature on clinical nutrition—both traditional and scientific—and modify my own diet and what I recommend for others based on that information. These recommendations have grown out of the answers I've found, both in study and in clinical experience, to four great questions in nutrition:

1. Why do primitive people who eat a traditional diet not suffer from the Western diseases?

2. Why do the Japanese have the longest life expectancy and the lowest rate of heart disease of all the developed countries?

3. Why do the French, who eat plenty of red meat and slather their foods with butter, cream, eggs, and rich pâtés, live almost as long as the Japanese, and have the second lowest heart attack rate in the world?

4. Why did our ancestors in the U.S. in 1900 suffer from a very low rate of heart disease, while it is our number one killer today?

Traditional Diets

I discussed the diets of various groups of indigenous people at length in Chapter 2. The most important factors in these diets seem to be no sugar, no processed foods, a high intake of minerals and trace elements, and a high intake—more than ten times what we take in today—of the fat-soluble vitamins A, D, and E. The table "Nutrients in Traditional Diets Compared to 20th Century Western Diets," from research by Weston Price, shows the mineral and vitamin density of some of these diets.

Japanese Diets

The Japanese live on average about four years longer than Americans. They also have dramatically lower rates of heart attacks and some cancers. If you want to cut your risk of heart attack by 80 percent and your risk of breast cancer by 70 percent, you might want to start eating like the Japanese (I'll describe how in the next chapter). Important factors in their diet may be high consumption of fish and other sea animals, high consumption of soy products, regular consumption of mineral-rich sea vegetables, and low consumption of sugar and processed foods.

NUTRIENTS IN TRADITIONAL DIETS COMPARED TO 20TH CENTURY WESTERN DIETS (NUMBERS REPRESENT PERCENTAGE GREATER IN TRADITIONAL DIETS)

	Calcium	Phosphorus	Magnesium	Iron	Fat-Soluble Vitamins
Eskimo	540%	500%	790%	150%	1,000+%
Swiss	370	220	250	310	1,000+
Gaelics	210	230	130	100	1,000+
Australian	460	620	170	5,060	1,000+
New Zealand Maori	620	690	2,340	5,830	1,000+
Melanesians	570	640	2,640	2,240	1,000+
Polynesians	560	720	2,850	1,860	1,000+
Peruvian Indians	660	550	1,360	510	1,000+
Africans (cattle raising)	750	820	1,910	1,660	1,000+
Africans (agricultural)	350	410	540	1,660	1,000+

(Source: Price, 1938)

THE FRENCH PARADOX

Some experts attribute the low rate of heart attacks in Japan—
the lowest in the world—solely to the lowfat, high-fish diet
there. France has about 80 percent more heart attacks per
capita than the Japanese, but about one-third as many as the
United States. In the region of Gascony in France, where goose
and duck liver are dietary staples, the figure drops to match
that of the Japanese (Fallon, 1995). Researchers have dubbed
this phenomenon the "French Paradox."

Several dietary theories have been put forward to explain the French Paradox. Current research is investigating
possible beneficial substances contained in red wine. I've been
unable to find a single researcher who has suggested the obvious—that refined vegetable oils, which disrupt the balance of
essential fatty acids and give the blood an increased tendency to
clot, are more destructive than the fat-soluble vitamin-rich animal fats that have been an integral part of our diet since the
dawn of humanity. The French also eat more sugar and refined
foods than the Japanese. If you want to cut your heart attack
risk by two-thirds, start eating like the French, but omit the
sugar and refined foods.

THE AMERICAN DIET IN 1900

Heart attacks as a major cause of death are a twentieth-century
development. Our great-grandparents may have died of heart
disease in their elder years, but it was more often *not* from a
heart attack caused by the blockage of the coronary arteries. So
rare were heart attacks in 1900 that physicians at the turn of the
century often had never observed one in their entire careers.
Since the turn of the century, however, all forms of heart disease
have risen dramatically, becoming the leading cause of death in

the 1950s. The figure "Deaths from Heart Disease" charts this dramatic rise in the first half of this century. The rates of deaths from heart disease tripled from 1900 levels by 1960.

If you want to reduce your risk of death from heart disease by two-thirds, eat the way your ancestors did. People in 1900 — 85 percent of the population lived on farms then — ate plenty of cholesterol, butter, eggs, and meat. They also ate farm-fresh vegetables, fresh-cracked grains, and fresh-pressed oils — all of it unprocessed and what we would call "organic" today.

Whatever caused this dramatic rise in deaths resulting from heart disease has come from societal and dietary changes between 1900 and 1948. The most important changes are: the introduction of refined white flour on a large scale; the introduction of refined processed vegetable oils, margarine, and other hydrogenated oils; the industrialization of livestock pro-

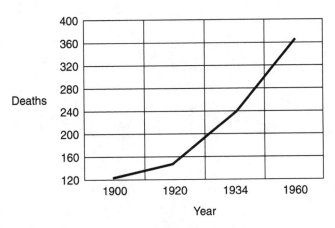

Deaths from heart disease per 100,000 U.S. population, 1900–1960. (Source: Price, 1938; USDC, 1997)

duction; and the demineralization of our soil and food (see Chapter 3).

It is my conclusion that the most important common health-giving factors are mineral density, richness in the fat soluble vitamins, and a balanced proportion of the essential fatty acids. Low fiber, high total-fat content, saturated fat, and cholesterol—the dietary factors emphasized as "negative" by the medical establishment today—may be important if you are eating a standard American diet, but fall away as disease-causing factors if you eat traditional whole foods, including high-quality meat, eggs, butter, and unprocessed organic whole grains, vegetables, and oils. I will discuss the myth of the benefits of the lowfat diet in more detail in Chapter 27.

CHAPTER 26

THE OPTIMUM MINERAL-RICH DIET

Can dietary changes cure disease? Although scientific evidence is plentiful to prove the ill effects of modern foods on health, evidence to prove the beneficial effects of a more healthful diet is scanty at best. Modern medicine, the driving force behind scientific medical research, does not employ diet therapy. Research scientists today are busy instead investigating drugs and the drug-like effects of single nutrients or occasionally single herbs. The standard of proof for modern medical science—the double-blind clinical trial—is impossible to conduct with total diet changes. The patient who makes sweeping changes in his or her diet will automatically know he or she did not receive a placebo. The contemporary scientific model also demands that a single controlled factor be studied. However, each individual making dietary changes will naturally select a somewhat different diet according to taste and preference. Although the new diet will have common factors—the addition of whole foods in their natural state and the removal of refined sugar, oils, and flours—neither the starting diet nor the new diet will be identical.

Thus we are left with epidemiological surveys and trials of single substances as our standard of science. Epidemiological studies and clinical trials of single foods or nutrients produce weak evidence at best because they do not take into account interactions of the single nutrients with the rest of the diet. A high-fat diet in one society, composed of one type of fats and oils taken along with highly processed foods, may have a completely different effect than a high-fat diet of natural fats and oils taken with whole foods in their natural state. It is thus impossible to prove, using modern scientific standards, that a nutrient-rich diet of foods in their natural state will cure disease. The best we can do is look at the general health of people and societies who consume such a diet, as Weston Price did in the 1930s, and try to model it. Even then, we cannot *prove* that adopting that diet will cure disease.

I have studied nature cure, and to some extent, formal naturopathic medicine, since 1973. During that time I have seen at least a thousand people who, after changing to a whole-foods diet, felt that they had been "raised from the dead." Some were not that sick to begin with. Others have had serious illnesses such as autoimmune diseases and cancer. Most of the cancer patients had already undergone some conventional treatment and modified their diets to prevent a recurrence or to avoid the chemotherapy that often follows surgical treatment. I have *never* seen a client who was willing to move toward a whole-foods diet whose health did not improve.

My experience matches that of nature cure practitioners in Western countries for at least the last 150 years. Within this healing tradition, the evidence is anecdotal—based on a large number of unique cases. But such evidence, if collected within a medical tradition, is not necessarily unscientific. It is, in fact, similar to the scientific support for modern surgical procedures. Surgical operations cannot be measured by double-blind methods either. No federal regulatory body requires proof of either safety or efficacy of surgical procedures. Instead, the body of knowledge of surgery is developed within the profession, based on anecdotal evidence and professional collaboration and communication, just like the diet therapies in nature cure.

MAKING CHANGES

Among my clients I find three attitudes toward dietary changes. Some people are ready to make a radical overhaul of their diets. Others are willing to make only gradual changes, or to change a few items in their diet. And some are unwilling to make any changes at all. I tell those in the last group that I will work with them, using mainly herbal remedies, but that I won't be able to help them much in the long run unless they improve their diets. I include mineral-rich beverage teas in their treatments. Fortunately, many of these people, after feeling some improvement as a result of the herbal treatments, are then willing to make some dietary changes. Most of my clients are in the second group and usually make long-term progress only in proportion to the dietary changes they make. Those in the first group invariably do best, provided they have a *genuine desire* for the dietary overhaul. If not, they usually soon feel deprived. If they can persist with the changes for six or eight weeks, they usually feel so much better that they will not return to their old ways of eating. Here are some tips for making changes in your diet:

> **First stage:** Start with healthy additions, without taking away anything that you currently enjoy.
>
> **Second stage:** Make some substitutions, such as mineral-rich sweeteners instead of sugar; homemade instead of canned soups; fresh-cooked grains and vegetables instead of processed ones; high-quality meats, organ

meats, and fish instead of packaged supermarket meats.

Third stage: Eliminate some unhealthy foods and addictions. This will be a lot easier if you have already made some of the changes listed previously and are feeling their benefits.

Fourth stage: Don't be fanatic. The nineteenth-century German naturopath Heinrich Lahmann said, "It's not what you eat on Sunday that matters, it's what you eat the other six days." He would prepare nice feasts of "stimulating" foods for the patients in his spa one day a week. Our physiology can handle feasting as long as it is not every day. And our spirits demand it occasionally.

SUGAR

Weston Price, and Burkitt and Trowell after him, identified sugar as a major culprit in the development of Western diseases. Slow dietary changes, with healthy additions and substitutions, are a wise course, but one food you can eliminate immediately to boost your health is refined sugar in all its forms (see Boxes 26.1 and 26.2). You will probably have to eliminate most canned and processed foods and soft drinks to do so. Most of the sugar we consume—about 85 percent—comes from sugar hidden in food. Ketchup contains about 50 percent sugar. McDonald's french fries contain about 20 percent sugar. Even cigarettes have 17 percent sugar in them.

In one scientific study, three ounces of sucrose eaten in one sitting reduced the ability of white blood cells to engulf bacteria and other invaders by about 40 percent. The effect started within a half hour and lasted more than five hours (Sanchez et al., 1973, and Ringsdorf et al., 1976). Another trial showed that

---

BOX 26.1

HIDDEN SUGAR IN YOUR FOOD

Here's a list of some of the names for sugars that may appear on the labels of processed foods. All are immuno-suppressive in the amounts consumed by the average American.

Barley malt	Invert sugar
Beet sugar	Lactose
Brown sugar	Levulose
Cane sugar	Maltose
Corn syrup	Milk sugar
Date sugar	Rice syrup
Dextrose	Succinate
Fructose	Sucrose
High-fructose corn syrup	Turbinado sugar
Honey	

---

only two ounces of glucose suppressed the activity of B- and T-lymphocytes, key components of immunity (Bernstein, 1977). Fructose, which was touted in the 1980s as a "healthy" sugar, actually depresses immunity even more (Appleton, 1997). Our average intake of 150 pounds of sugar per year adds up to more than six ounces a day—three times the level necessary to depress the immune system. A single soft drink may contain two ounces of sugar.

A clinical trial into the relationship between sugar and cavities demonstrates sugar's devastating systemic effects. Researchers fed people sugar through a tube so it would bypass their teeth and mouth. They found that the flow of a saliva-like

---

BOX 26.2

SOME OF THE ADVERSE EFFECTS OF SUGAR

Suppression of the immune system

Reduction of calcium and magnesium absorption

Exhaustion of the body's chromium supplies

Mineral depletion of bones and tissues

Reduction of high-density lipoproteins ("good" cholesterol)

Elevation of low-density lipoproteins ("bad" cholesterol)

Elevation of serum triglycerides

Tooth and gum disease

Contribution to many of the Western diseases shown in Table 2.8

(Source: Appleton, 1997)

---

liquid from the gums, which normally washes food particles away from the teeth, reversed its flow and began sucking food particles against the border of the gums and teeth instead (Appleton, 1997). The decay-inducing effects of sugar are not caused by sugar on the tooth surface but from system-wide reactions to the presence of sugar.

Virtually every tissue in the body is adversely affected. For an exhaustive review of the scientific literature on sugar, see *Lick the Sugar Habit* by Nancy Appleton (1996). Appleton spent more than ten years reviewing the scientific literature on sugar before writing her book, and she includes complete scientific references on its adverse effects. She concludes that sugar has an addictive drug-like effect on some people, and she also gives tips for quitting the habit. See Figure 26.1 for an x-ray of

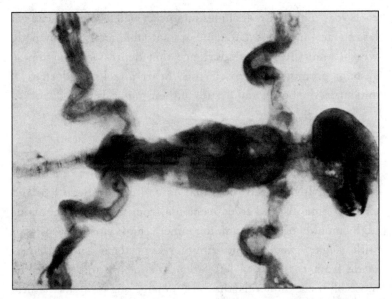

Figure 26.1 Shown is the grossly demineralized and deformed skeleton of a pet monkey fed on sweets and pastries. (Photos and caption reprinted from Price, 1938.)

the skeleton of a pet monkey that had been fed only pastries and sweets. The sugar in the pastry completely deformed the skeleton by robbing its minerals.

Consumption

The average American consumes about 150 pounds of sugar and corn syrup a year (U.S. Department of Commerce, 1996), with about twenty-six pounds of that coming from soft drinks. A typical soft drink contains about fifteen tablespoons of sugar, and the average American drinks 557 of them a year. That number has more than doubled since 1970. Americans on average consume the weight of a typical adult body in sugar each year. This figure includes infants as well as people who eat less sugar—meaning that some of us double or triple our body weight annually with a substance that depresses the immune system; promotes atherosclerosis, heart attacks, and strokes; and strips the bones and tissues of their minerals.

Substitutes

Sugarcane, the source of refined white sugar, is a mineral-rich plant. It has deep roots that extend up to fifteen feet and extract minerals and trace elements from the soil. It contains high amounts of chromium, the mineral most closely associated with sugar metabolism. Another sweetener—molasses—is made from the residue left after refinement, and it contains most of those minerals that accompany sugar in its natural state. A small amount of molasses added to the sugar makes brown sugar. Blackstrap molasses is highly concentrated sugarcane juice and tastes nowhere near as sweet as sugar. Table 26.1 shows the comparative mineral value of sugarcane derivatives. I've included honey in the chart to show how closely it resembles white sugar. Many people eat honey instead of sugar, thinking that it is "healthy," when actually it contains less mineral nutrition than even brown sugar. Although honey does contain more of a few trace elements than white or brown sugar, it is a mineral-depleting food. Eat it the way traditional people did—on special occasions.

Blackstrap molasses may not taste so sweet, but it is one of the best mineral supplements we have. A tablespoon of it—three times the amount shown in Table 26.1—contains up to one-third of the minimum daily requirement of some of the minerals and trace elements. British natural healer Cyril Scott used blackstrap molasses to cure a wide variety of mineral-deficiencies earlier in this century. His classic work *Crude Black*

TABLE 26.1   MINERALS IN FOOD PRODUCTS
FROM SUGARCANE
(MILLIGRAMS PER 1 TEASPOON)

	White Sugar	Honey	Brown Sugar	Regular Molasses	Blackstrap Molasses
Calcium	0.042	0.38	3.91	13.66	57.33
Iron	0.003	0.27	0.088	0.315	1.17
Magnesium	0	0.13	1.3	16.13	14.33
Phosphorus	0.084	0.25	1.0	2.17	2.67
Potassium	0.084	3.27	15.9	97.6	166.0
Zinc	0.001	0.014	0.008	0.019	0.067
Copper	0.002	0.002	0.014	0.032	0.136
Manganese	0	0.005	0.015	0.101	0.174

Molasses was reprinted by Benedict Lust Publications in 1980 and is still available in book stores today. Keep molasses, and especially blackstrap molasses, on your table and use it in place of sugars, jellies, and jams. Add it to soups, breads, juices, and other drinks.

RED MEAT

Now that I've told you to take something out of your diet, let's look at a food category you can keep. Contemporary nutritionists advise that we reduce our intake of red meat. Yet Weston Price observed that many traditional societies ate red meat and enjoyed near-perfect health. Our ancestors in 1900 also ate plenty of it and suffered far fewer heart attacks than we do today. Red meat is a healthful food, if taken in the context of an otherwise mineral- and vitamin-rich whole-foods diet and not taken in great excess. The saturated fats in red meat may cause problems in the absence of the mineral and vitamin antioxidants and essential fatty acids frequently missing from our diets.

Beef

Red meat itself is not a "bad" food, but the beef we find in our supermarkets today may be unhealthy. Our cattle have been bred to be fat. The cattle of the Masai and related tribes in Africa are lean with a fat profile resembling that of the wild game animals in Table 2.7 (Erasmus, 1993). Selectively bred cattle in the United States today have four to ten times the fat content of beef as it naturally occurs. Most cattle in America today are also raised in feedlots. They are not allowed to graze on their natural diet of grasses, but are fed prepared foods and demineralized grains to fatten them up. Many become so sickly that they need antibiotics to stay alive, and these antibiotic residues can remain in the meat. Cattle also often receive steroid drugs for weight gain. Changes in cattle breeding and feeding have also eliminated the vitamin A content in beef during the last thirty years (see Table 3.12). Plenty of vitamin A remains in beef organ meats, which I'll discuss following.

You may not be able to get wild African beef in America today, but you can get the sort of beef that our ancestors ate in 1900. Many larger natural food stores now carry meat from grass-fed cows and other animals that are allowed to roam their pastures and rangeland and eat their natural diets. The meat is also free of antibiotics and steroid hormones. I've been unable to find nutrient analyses on such meats, but the animals are surely healthier, their essential fatty acids (which come from eating green plants) higher, and their minerals and trace elements higher than animals fed mineral-depleted corn. You could also buy sides of beef directly from a farmer and freeze it.

Lamb

The contemporary scientific studies that show red meat to be bad for you invariably lump feedlot-raised beef and pork together with lamb in a single category. The way these animals are raised, however, is very different. Most of the lamb meat you buy in stores today comes from animals that are grass-fed, rather than artificially fed with fattening, mineral-deficient foods and drugs in feedlots. Lamb has almost 20 percent less fat and about 15 percent less sodium than beef, both positive changes for the American public. The fat content in lamb is also much higher in essential fatty acids than beef, with lamb having a similar percentage of EFAs to that in bison (see Table 2.7). Its levels of omega-3 fatty acids, which is responsible for some of the health benefits of fish and wild game, is in the same range as that of some fish (see Table 26.3). Although lamb contains slightly less iron, it contains about 17 percent more of the trace elements measured. Presumably this increase applies to other essential trace elements as well. The lamb also contains 70 percent more vitamins in the B complex. Lamb may not be as high quality a meat as wild game, but is much healthier than beef.

I would not suggest eating lamb or other red meat every day, and I recommend against eating any supermarket beef at all, but you don't need to eliminate red meat completely to stay healthy.

Organ Meats

Healthy meat eaters of the past—both traditional people and our more recent European ancestors—did not eat the muscle meat of animals alone. They also ate the organ meats. Some people considered them the choicest part of the animal. Weston Price found that Northern Canadian Indians ate the internal organs and bone marrow of deer and fed the muscle meat to their dogs. The Hebrides Islanders' favorite dish was fish head (complete with the brains) stuffed with fish livers. This trend was found in most of the traditional peoples Price studied. Organ meats are also a traditional food of many of our European ancestors. As I was growing up in a family of mostly Irish extraction, we had liver once a week. A friend of Italian extraction tells me that her grandparents still eat brains once a week. Table 26.2 shows the nutrient values of some of today's supermarket organ meats. Liver contains huge quantities of trace elements and fat-soluble vitamins. You don't need to eat these foods every day. A once-a-week serving provides a good nutrition boost. If you are not used to organ meats, you'll have to develop a taste for them. I recommend the book *Nourishing Tra-*

TABLE 26.2   NUTRIENTS IN SOME ORGAN MEATS (PER 100 GRAMS OF MEAT)

Nutrient	Beef Liver	Chicken Liver	Beef Kidney
Protein	20 g	17.97 g	16.88 g
Fat	3.85 g	3.86 g	21.95 g
Iron	6.82 mg	8.56 mg	1.57 mg
Zinc	3.92 mg	3.07 mg	3.33 mg
Copper	3.339 mg	0.395 mg	0.104 mg
Manganese	0.264 mg	0.258 mg	0.019 mg
Thiamin	0.26 mg	0.138 mg	0.12 mg
Riboflavin	2.78 mg	1.963 mg	0.22 mg
Niacin	12.78 mg	9.25 mg	6.1 mg
Pantothenic acid	7.62 mg	6.184 mg	0.67 mg
Vitamin B$_6$	0.94 mg	0.76 mg	0.13 mg
Folate	248 mcg	738 mcg	18 mcg
Vitamin B$_{12}$	69.19 mcg	22.98 mcg	2.39 mcg
Vitamin A	35,346 IU	20,549 IU	0

(Source: U.S. Department of Agriculture, 1997)

ditions by Sally Fallon, which contains a number of recipes and shopping tips for organ meats. The book contains more than seven hundred recipes for a variety of foods, based in part on the work of Weston Price. The organ meats of grass-fed, hormone- and antibiotic-free animals are available in many natural food stores today.

FISH

If you pick only one meat to add to your diet to improve your health, it should be fish. Hundreds of clinical studies have shown that fish and fish oil can improve cardiovascular health and reduce inflammation in chronic diseases. One of the reasons the Japanese are healthier than the people of other developed countries is that they eat a lot of fish. Probably the most beneficial substance in fish is the omega-3 fatty acid called eicosapentaenoic acid, or EPA. EPA, which reduces both inflammation and the tendency of the blood to form clots, also occurs abundantly in wild game such as deer and elk. Table 26.3 shows a nutrient comparison of the omega-3 fatty acids and other nutrients in fish and a variety of meats. Notice that not all fish have a high percentage of omega-3 fatty acids. Cod, canned tuna, and bass fall near the bottom of the list. Notice also that farmed salmon falls in between retail cuts of beef and ground beef. Farmed fish are kept in a pool—the equivalent of cattle feedlots—and fed prepared foods. They are not allowed to roam the seas or streams and eat the omega-3-rich green foods that make up their natural diet. Their fat profile then resembles that of beef raised and fed in a similar manner.

Much of the fish available in supermarkets today is farmed fish and does not have the health benefits of wild varieties. If you find "Atlantic salmon" in a store today, it is probably farmed in the fisheries of New England. If you select your

TABLE 26.3   PERCENTAGE OF OMEGA-3
FATTY ACIDS IN FISH AND MEATS
(PER 100 GRAMS OF MEAT)

Food	Total Fat (Grams)	Omega-3 Fatty Acids (%)
Salmon (wild)	6.34	4.65
Salmon (cooked)	8.13	4.60
Sardines (canned)	11.45	4.35
Trout	3.46	3.44
Halibut	2.29	2.84
Deer	2.42	2.89
Elk	1.45	2.76
Catfish	2.82	2.52
Lamb	21.59	1.81
Bison (wild)	1.84	1.63
Beef (retail cuts)	19.20	1.19
Salmon (canned)	6.05	0.95
Chicken	15.06	0.93
Salmon (farmed)	10.85	0.87
Shrimp	1.73	0.81
Beefalo	4.8	0.80
Bass	2.33	0.64
Pork (retail cuts)	14.95	0.60
Beef (ground)	26.55	0.60
Clams	0.97	0.41
Snapper	1.34	0.30
Tuna (canned)	0.82	0.20
Shrimp (fast food)	15.10	0.17
Cod	0.67	0.15

meats from bison—the lowest of the game meats in the table—
and above, you will be imitating the natural diets of the primitive people that Weston Price studied. Notice that although
lamb falls within that range, the fish at the top of the list have
more than three times the percentage of omega-3 oils.

OILS

The introduction of refined oils to the American diet in the first decades of this century has probably contributed to our dramatic rise in atherosclerosis and heart disease. The main culprits are refined vegetable oils and margarine and related hydrogenated oils and shortenings. Our ancestors in the last century consumed oils, but they were invariably fresh-pressed oils that easily became rancid and were marketed as perishable foods like milk or eggs. These oils were rich in many of the nutrients in the original plant being pressed. Table 26.4 shows the steps of refinement of oils today. These refined oils, or even the so-called "unrefined oils" you might find in a health food store, are depleted of the vitamins, minerals, and other substances that occur naturally in the plant. Their effects in the body are similar to those of white sugar or white flour. To metabolize their calories, the body must rob the bones and tissues of their stored nutrients.

Besides their mineral-stripping effects, the massive increase of vegetable oils, margarine, and shortening in our society has created an imbalance in tissue levels of our essential fatty acids. Fatty acid biochemistry is very complex. If you are interested in very thorough information on the subject, I suggest the book *Fats That Heal, Fats That Kill* by Udo Erasmus, Ph.D. The best brief explanation I've found on the topic, with full scientific references, is contained in the chapter on oils in the *Encyclopedia of Nutritional Supplements* by Michael Murray, N.D. I'll give a capsule summary here.

The two classes of essential fatty acids we require in our diets are omega-3 and omega-6 oils. Most vegetable oils are highest in the omega-6 oils. We must have these oils to maintain our health—they are even present in mother's milk. The omega-6 oils are converted into two different kinds of prostaglandins, hormone-like substances with powerful effects on our cells. The

TABLE 26.4 STEPS IN THE REFINEMENT OF VEGETABLE OILS

Stage	Description	Nutrients	By-product or Product
Raw material	Seeds, nuts, beans	Oils, protein, minerals, vitamins, fiber	
Step 1	Clean and hull	No effect	
Step 2	Add solvent	Lose protein, fiber, vitamins, minerals	Product: "Unrefined oil"
Step 3	Distill and degum	Lose chlorophyll, calcium, magnesium, copper, iron	By-product: Lecithin
Step 4	Refine	Lose phospholipids, minerals	
Step 5	Bleach	Lose chlorophyll, beta-carotene, flavor compounds	
Step 6	Deodorize	Lose vitamin E	By-product: Vitamin E
Step 7	Add preservatives		Product: Supermarket oil
Step 8	Hydrogenate	Lose essential fatty acids	Product: Margarine and shortening

(Source: Erasmus, 1993)

series-1 prostaglandins from omega-6 oils are anti-inflammatory and have a wide range of other healthy effects. Series-2 prostaglandins, on the other hand, are inflammatory and increase the tendency of our blood to clot. The body prefers to make series-1 prostaglandins out of dietary omega-6 oils and, with a healthy natural diet, only makes enough of the series-2 prostaglandins to maintain a healthy inflammatory response to infections and irritants. Drugs like aspirin and corticosteroids act by suppressing the effects of these series-2 prostaglandins. Aspirin also blocks the blood clot–promoting effects of these prostaglandins, which is why doctors tell people who have had heart attacks to take an aspirin every other day.

We also require a third kind of prostaglandin, the series-3 prostaglandins from omega-3 oils, which are also anti-inflammatory and have other health benefits. The body, in its wisdom, has the ability to launch an inflammatory response, but has two substances—series-1 and series-3 prostaglandins—that will control and moderate that response so it does not get out of hand. These three substances have to be in balance. If we get our omega-3 oils from fish or wild game, it comes in the form of EPA (see previous discussion of fish), which is readily converted into the series-3 prostaglandins. If we don't eat fish or wild game, and eat meat from domesticated livestock that contains only low amounts of these oils, our body has a mechanism to covert alpha-linolenic acid, an omega-3 oil in some plant foods, into EPA. Alpha-linolenic acid is present in small amounts in many oils, but is highest in hemp seed oil, flaxseed oil, canola oil, and soy oil (in highest to lowest order of content). Alpha-linolenic acid is contained in green plants, but only in low amounts. This is where the fish and wild game obtain it, and we require such an animal intermediary to concentrate enough from greens to be of use to us.

This conversion from alpha-linolenic to EPA acid is complex and can be blocked by a number of deficiencies or excesses, including:

- vitamin B$_6$ deficiency
- vitamin C deficiency
- magnesium deficiency
- zinc deficiency
- fatty acids from margarine or shortening
- excess oils containing omega-6 fatty acids

The fatty acids in margarine and shortening have been chemically manipulated to make solid an oil that would normally be liquid at room temperature. The result is a fat molecule that is completely foreign to the human body. Scientific studies of the effect of these substances on heart disease have been contradictory—margarine-eaters in some societies have higher incidence of heart disease, and in others they have lower incidence of heart disease. This may be due to other factors in the national diets of those countries. However, it makes common sense not to consume such an unnatural substance, especially when it is known to interfere with the normal metabolism of alpha-linolenic acid.

We saw in Chapter 4 that both men and women in the United States are on average deficient in magnesium and zinc. Vitamin B$_6$ and vitamin C are also commonly deficient (Werbach, 1993). We consume large amounts of margarine and related oils, often hidden in processed foods. And we consume large amounts of the oils containing omega-6. Table 26.5 outlines the results this has on the oil balance in our tissues. When the conversion of alpha-linolenic acid is inhibited through malnutrition, the enzymes that would normally produce EPA from alpha-linolenic acid instead begin to affect the omega-6 pathway so that the body produces more inflammatory series-2

Table 26.5   Percentage of Essential Fatty
Acids in Human Body Fat
(1991–1992)

Society	% Omega-6	% Omega-3	Ratio
New Zealand Maori	2.6	0.93	2.8:1
Japanese	14.8	3.2	4.6:1
American	10.2	0.58	17.6:1

(Source: Erasmus, 1993)

prostaglandins. We get an increase of the inflammatory, blood-thickening, series-2 prostaglandins and a deficiency of the anti-inflammatory prostaglandins of series-3. It is a social formula for inflammatory diseases, heart attacks, and strokes. It is my opinion that the imbalance of our dietary oils, especially the high consumption of vegetable oils and margarine, coupled with the demineralization of our soil and foods, account for the dramatic rise in heart disease in the United States in this century.

The huge imbalance in the omega-6 to omega-3 ratio in Americans results from low consumption of wild fish and game with corresponding high consumption of EPA-deficient commercial livestock and poultry; high consumption of refined omega-6 oils; high consumption of margarine; and common vitamin and mineral deficiencies.

The natural therapeutic diet for this condition would include: fish, game, and other meats high in EPA; reduction of refined omega-6 oils such as corn, peanut, and safflower oil, and eating more corn, safflowers, or peanuts instead; complete elimination of margarine and shortening, including that contained in processed foods; and eating whole, unprocessed, mineral- and vitamin-rich plant foods. A high-quality, broad-spectrum multiple vitamin and mineral supplement makes sense if disease is already present. For decades now, doctors have been telling people to eat margarine and vegetable oils instead of animal fats, but the animal fats are actually better for you because they do not disrupt the essential fatty acid metabolism the way vegetable oils do.

OLIVE OIL

A natural substitute for the omega-6 processed vegetable oils is virgin olive oil. It contains only low levels of omega-3 or omega-6 oils, so it will not interfere with prostaglandin production or balance. No saturated fat appears in virgin oils, so for cardiovascular health they are "neutral." Olive oil also does not oxidize—turn rancid—very easily and keeps well at room temperature. Virgin olive oil is by definition made from high-quality olives by simple pressing.

Extra-virgin olive oil is made from even higher quality olives. The olive-quality standards (but not the pressing method) for virgin oil were reduced in the last decade, so an extra-virgin oil today equals the virgin oil of the past. Virgin oils contain most of the nutrient elements that you see removed during refining in Table 26.4. Olive oil that is refined, rather than virgin, falls in the same nutrient-deficient category as the other refined oils.

Although the oil content of virgin oil has a neutral effect on cardiovascular health, it also contains a number of other substances, listed in table 26.6, that may be beneficial to the heart. I removed all margarine from my diet and began using olive oils exclusively about twenty years ago, and, at age fifty, have no allergies or other inflammatory conditions (even though the rest of my family of origin is allergy prone), and lab tests show a low likelihood of atherosclerosis. I recommend that you purchase the highest quality olive oil you can find, which usually means it's the most expensive.

TABLE 26.6   SOME BENEFICIAL SUBSTANCES
IN VIRGIN OLIVE OILS

Substance	Effect
Beta-carotene	Antioxidant
Vitamin E	Antioxidant
Chlorophyll (contains magnesium)	Nourishes the heart
Squalene	Protects the heart
Phytosterols	Reduce cholesterol

EGGS

Eggs were unfortunately tagged as a "bad" food several decades ago when the theory that dietary cholesterol causes heart disease was popular among scientists. The simplest refutation of this theory is that heart attacks were rare in 1900, and common today, but dietary cholesterol has remained about constant during that time. The Japanese also consume more cholesterol than Americans do, and they have a very low rate of heart disease.

Almost all the cholesterol in the body is produced by the liver and does not come from the diet. Most people who take in more dietary cholesterol simply produce less from their liver to compensate. Even the link between high cholesterol and heart disease has been questioned in the last few years. It seems that high cholesterol itself is not the culprit, but rather oxidized cholesterol. The cause of atherosclerosis is whatever initially injures the arteries to initiate plaque formation, whatever oxidizes the cholesterol, and a deficiency of antioxidant vitamins and minerals. Refined and cooked vegetable oils are highly oxidative and are a logical suspect for the oxidative injuries to the vessels and the oxidation of cholesterol. I will discuss some questionable myths about the value of lowfat diets in Chapter

27. The quality and type of fat is more important than the amount.

Eggs are rich in nutrients, especially the fat-soluble vitamins A and D. Table 26.7 shows the nutrients in a cooked, three-egg omelet, with and without whole-milk Cheddar cheese. Organic eggs, from chickens that are allowed to move around and feed on natural grasses, contain omega-6 and omega-3 oils in about a 1:1 ratio—close to the ideal balance. Some supermarket eggs may contain almost twenty times more omega-6 than omega-3 oils (Simopaulus and Salem, 1992). The shells of free-range chicken eggs are much thicker—you have to hit them harder to break them—indicating that the chickens are healthier and have a higher mineral content in their diet.

MILK AND MILK PRODUCTS

Cow's or goat's milk is a traditional food in some parts of the world, especially in cold climates with long winters, but is not consumed at all in most areas. Many Asians, Africans, and

TABLE 26.7 NUTRIENTS IN A
THREE-EGG OMELET

	Eggs Only	With Whole-Milk Cheddar Cheese (3 ounces)
Protein	30.99 g	55.89 g
Fat	34.32 g	67.42 g
Calcium	76.86 mg	798.16 mg
Potassium	184.8 mg	553.2 mg
Iron	2.19 mg	2.87 mg
Zinc	1.683 mg	4.793 mg
Vitamin A	1,197 IU	2,256 IU
Vitamin D	1.8 mcg	2.7 mcg
Vitamin E	2.361 IU	2.601 IU

people descended from them cannot tolerate dairy foods at all. Digestion of milk sugar requires an enzyme called *lactase*, which some races and individuals lack. Babies naturally produce this enzyme, but it disappears after weaning. Milk protein — called *casein* — is also difficult to digest and is perceived by the immune system of some individuals as if it were part of a bacterium or virus. Those people who can tolerate milk best seem to be those descended from cultural groups that have consumed a lot of it. All traditional people who consume milk also make fermented milk products, such as yogurt and buttermilk. This process predigests the milk protein and makes it easier to assimilate. Cheese contains highly concentrated milk protein, and those who are sensitive to milk should avoid cheese completely. Cooking also makes cheese harder to digest.

Milk allergy is the most common food sensitivity in the United States, followed by wheat. I once interviewed the head of an ear, nose, and throat department in a major teaching hospital on the topic of childhood ear infections. He received many referrals from general practitioners to surgically place tubes in the children's ears. He told me that he could prevent about 25 percent of the surgeries by screening for cow's milk allergies. When the children stopped consuming milk and milk products, their ear infections went away. When a person consumes milk, or any other food allergen, it evokes a powerful immune response in the gut. The circulating white blood cells drop by about 40 percent as they rush to the site of the irritation. This leaves other areas of the body deficient, and infections of the tonsils, sinuses, and ears may set in. My clinical experience with sinus infections is not very extensive, but to date I have never seen a chronic sinus infection in a person who did not drink milk. Many of the infections cleared up by removing milk and cheese from the diet. I had one patient who had suffered life-long infections and immune disorders, including fungal infection in infancy, childhood eczema, upper respiratory infections, urinary tract infections, and, finally, systemic lupus, an autoimmune disease. She had been fed cow's milk too early in infancy, before her gut could handle it, and the lifelong dairy overload had wreaked havoc on her immune system. Immediate removal of dairy products put a halt to her most serious lupus symptoms. Most people who are allergic to dairy can eat butter, which does not contain either the casein or the lactose, without repercussions. Very sensitive people who can't tolerate even butter can eat ghee (clarified butter), which has all milk solids removed. Beware of inexpensive ghee in imported food stores, however—it usually contains vegetable oils and margarine that are not listed on the label.

Whole raw milk is delivered by the mother animal in a state that is ideal for its digestion and assimilation. This includes not only vitamins and minerals, but also enzymes that assist in their assimilation. Unfortunately, the modern processes of pasteurization and homogenization destroy these enzymes, and milk processed this way is even more difficult to digest than milk in its natural state. Calves fed pasteurized milk develop joint stiffness and do not thrive. Why should we drink milk that makes a baby cow sick?

Raw milk is still obtainable through health food stores in some states, but other states have banned it as a health hazard, because of occasional outbreaks of salmonella food poisoning. It is ironic that the vast majority of salmonella outbreaks have occurred from pasteurized rather than raw milk. One such outbreak in Illinois affected more than 14,000 people, including two who died (Fallon, 1995). Raw goat's milk is also available in many areas, and has a significantly higher concentration of trace elements than commercial cow's milk (see Table 26.8).

Milk fat is one of the most nutritious sources of fat available to humans. It is rich in vitamin A, and its essential fatty acid balance is ideal, about 1:1 omega-6 to omega-3 fatty acids. Unfortunately our society is now in "anti-fat" mode, and sales

TABLE 26.8   SOME NUTRIENTS IN
              PASTEURIZED WHOLE COW'S
              MILK VS. GOAT'S MILK

	Cow	Goat	% Increase
Protein	8 g	8.6 g	7.50
Fat	8.9 g	10.1 g	13.48
Calcium	290.3 g	325 g	11.95
Potassium	368.4 g	498 g	35.18
Zinc	0.927 mg	0.732 mg	−21.04
Copper	0.024 mg	0.112 mg	366.67
Manganese	0.01 mg	0.044 mg	340.00
Vitamin A	336.7 IU	451.4 IU	34.07

of butter, whole milk, and cheese have declined dramatically in favor of lowfat varieties. In the process of cutting the fat in milk and related products from about 4 percent to about 2 percent, about half the beneficial elements in the fat are also cut. Box 26.3 shows some of the nutrients in butter. Eating more butter

---

BOX 26.3

NUTRIENTS IN BUTTER (1 TABLESPOON)

Fat: 11.5 g
Saturated fat: 7.1 g
Omega-6 fatty acids: 0.26 mg
Omega-3 fatty acids: 0.17 mg
Percent EFA: 3.74%
Vitamin A: 434 IU
Vitamin D: 0.3 mcg

(Source: USDA, 1997)

TABLE 26.9   SOME BENEFICIAL
                       CONSTITUENTS IN BUTTER

Benefit	Description
Wulzen (anti-stiffness) factor	Protects against degenerative arthritis, hardening of the arteries, and cataracts
Short- and medium-chains fatty acids	About 15 percent of butterfat. Absorbed directly by the small intestine without emulsification by the bile. Antimicrobial, anti-tumor, immune stimulating, antifungal
Conjugated linoleic acid	Anticancer
Glycosphingolipids	Protect against gastrointestinal infections
Trace minerals	Chromium, iodine, manganese, selenium, and zinc

(Source: Fallon, 1995)

fat and less vegetable oils and margarine would shift the essential fatty acid balance in your body toward that of the Japanese and the traditional Australian aborigines, both of which are unusually healthy cultures. High butter consumption among the French, with this balance of fatty acids, may partly explain the French Paradox (see section introduction). Butter also contains other beneficial constituents (see Table 26.9). Table 26.10 shows the nutrients that are lost in lowfat cheese compared to whole milk cheese.

SOY PRODUCTS

Soy products are among the most popular foods in Japan and other parts of Asia, and researchers think that soy consumption

TABLE 26.10   SOME NUTRIENTS IN WHOLE
VS. LOWFAT CHEDDAR CHEESE
(PER 100 GRAMS OF CHEESE)

Nutrient	Whole	Lowfat	% Change
Protein	24.9 g	24.35 g	–2.21
Fat	33.1 g	7 g	–78.85
Calcium	721.3 g	415 g	–42.46
Potassium	368.4 g	66 g	–82.08
Iron	0.68 g	0.42 g	–38.24
Zinc	3.11 mg	1.82 mg	–41.48
Copper	0.031 mg	0.021 mg	–32.26
Manganese	0.01 mg	0.006 mg	–40.00
Vitamin A	1059 IU	233 IU	–78.00
Vitamin E	0.24 IU	0.079 IU	–67.08
Essential fatty acids	0.942 g	0.223 g	–76.33

contributes to the superior health and longevity of the Japanese. Soy is rich in minerals and essential fatty acids. It also contains hormone-like substances that can reduce the intensity of menopausal symptoms. Table 26.11 lists some of the nutrients in soy products. Tempeh, my personal favorite soy food, is made from fermented and aged soybeans. Although levels of some of the minerals in tempeh appear lower than those in tofu, the minerals are more bioavailable in tempeh. Tofu and other unfermented soy products, including the cooked beans, contain high levels of phytates, which bind some minerals and make them unavailable. Unfermented soy also contains enzyme-inhibiting substances that can impair digestion of all foods if consumed in large quantities. Another excellent fermented soy product is miso, a paste-like product that will dissolve easily in soups. Season tempeh any way you want, put it in casseroles, stir-fries, or traditional dishes such as spaghetti sauce or tacos. Vegetarians who eat tofu alone cannot expect to get the health

TABLE 26.11   MINERALS AND ESSENTIAL
FATTY ACIDS IN SOY PRODUCTS
(PER 100 GRAMS OF FOOD)*

Nutrient	Cooked Soybeans	Cooked Tofu	Cooked Tempeh
Calcium (mg)	102	205	93
Iron (mg)	5.14	10.47	2.26
Magnesium (mg)	86	94	70
Potassium (mg)	515	237	367
Zinc (mg)	1.15	1.57	1.81
Copper (mg)	0.407	0.378	0.67
Manganese (mg)	0.824	1.181	1.43
Total fat (g)	8.9	8.72	7.68
% Essential fatty acids	56.94	56.43	56.41
% Omega-3 fatty acids	6.72	6.67	6.67

*The minerals in cooked soybeans and tofu are bound to plant substances called phytates, which inhibit their absorption. The phytates are destroyed during the fermentation of tempeh

benefits of the Japanese, who eat it as a secondary food and not as a primary protein source. The Japanese consume their soy products along with fish and fish soup stocks.

GRAINS

We take white wheat flour so much for granted now that we think of it as a natural food. Refined flours, like refined sugar, not only deny you the nutrition available in the whole food, but rob the body of the vitamins and minerals necessary to digest and metabolize them. See Table 2.4 for a comparison of white versus whole wheat bread. In our supermarkets, white flour is almost always combined with sugar as well, making matters worse.

Traditional peoples in many areas of the world consume grains, but not in the forms we do today. Traditional cultures do

---

CASE STUDY #1

An elderly woman with multiple health problems, including constipation, fatigue, and rheumatoid arthritis, was reluctant to change her dietary habits. The simple addition of oatmeal for breakfast, and substitution of whole wheat bread for white bread, completely eliminated her constipation and improved the other problems within three weeks. No laxatives were given at all.

---

not eat bread! At least not without preparing the grains first by soaking and/or fermenting them. Our ancestors throughout Europe, Africa, South America, South Asia, and even the European colonists in America prepared their grains this way. Traditional Irish oatmeal is prepared by roasting whole oats, cracking or grinding them, soaking them overnight in water, and finally cooking them in the morning. Traditional Swiss muesli is made from fresh-cracked oats or other grains that are soaked overnight in water with a little live yogurt culture added and then cooked. Many traditional breads, including American sourdough bread, are made by letting the dough ferment before baking. This practice of traditional wisdom, in use for countless centuries before minerals were discovered, greatly improves the availability of minerals in grains. All grains, and many beans, contain phytic acid in their outer layers. Phytic acid binds minerals in the intestinal tract—especially zinc—and inhibits their absorption. Soaking grains, especially in an acid medium, destroys the phytic acid and frees the minerals for easy absorption. Fermenting grains also helps to predigest their proteins, reducing some of the work for the digestive tract.

Traditional peoples also usually crack their grains just before using, retaining all the nutrients as they exist in the living seed. You can plant a whole oat and it will grow. Try doing that with the rolled oats in commercial oatmeal, or with a handful of wheat flour. As soon as a grain is cracked, it begins losing nutrients, and any oils present begin to go rancid. Mineral content will remain the same, but vitamins degrade. My first job in the health foods business in 1973 was as a whole-grain baker for a sandwich shop. Each morning I took fresh wheat berries, ground them into flour, and turned them into bread within a few hours of cracking. You have to taste bread or oatmeal prepared this way to believe how delicious it is. Needless to say, our shop did a booming sandwich business. The fresh-cracked grains have a sweetness and vitality that is missing if the flour is allowed to sit for even twenty-four hours. I still fresh-grind my grains in a flour mill, but now I soak them overnight before making bread, oatmeal, porridge, or pancakes.

Wheat, corn, rye, barley, and oats all contain a protein called *gluten*. The gluten in kneaded wheat dough makes up the thick matrix that captures the gas from the fermenting yeast and makes wheat bread rise so nicely. Gluten is very hard to digest, and, for some of us, the immune system treats it as a foreign invader and mounts an allergic reaction against it. Infants and young children who are fed gluten-containing bread and grain products often develop a lifelong allergy to it. Wheat allergies are among the most common food allergies in the United States, second only to cow's milk. Gluten can cause some overt conditions such as celiac disease, irritable bowel syndrome, and ulcerative colitis. It can also cause less obvious symptoms such as depression, fatigue, weight gain, edema, and heightened tendency to airborne allergies. If you wonder whether you have a wheat allergy, try cutting out all gluten-containing grains for six weeks and see if any of your health problems go away. One clue

---

Case Study #2

A forty-four-year-old-man had experienced unexplainable weight gains over a period of five years. He exercised moderately and his diet appeared healthful, without sugar or excess fats or oils, but he had gained five to ten pounds a year during that period. The weight tended to come in spurts, sometimes as much a eight pounds in a month, and never went back to the lower weight. His morning body temperature had dropped eight-tenths of a degree during the same period, to 97.8. A hypothyroid condition could cause these symptoms, but his thyroid hormone levels were within normal limits. His diet diary revealed that he ate wheat most days. After six weeks of cutting out all wheat, including the wheat hidden in common processed foods, he had lost five pounds and his morning body temperature had risen a half a degree.

---

that you may have an allergy is if you tend to binge on a food or if you do not consider your day complete without it.

Of the five gluten-containing grains, oats have the lowest amount, and some people who cannot tolerate gluten can take oats without ill effect, especially if they are fermented with water and a little yogurt overnight. Rice, millet, and buckwheat, which do not contain gluten, are much less likely to cause food allergies. These grains also contain phytic acid, and their mineral nutrients will be more available if soaked overnight. Many Americans who have developed allergies to wheat and corn from being fed those grains too early in infancy tolerate these "foreign" grains quite well. Try putting a cup of brown rice with three cups of water in the top of a double boiler. Let it simmer over medium-low heat for four or five hours. The result is a very sweet rice with a consistency like white rice.

Fruits and Vegetables

We saw in Table 3.16 that organic fruits and vegetables have on average about twice the mineral content of supermarket varieties. Organic produce is also free of pesticides. Some people balk at the higher average prices for organic produce, but if you figure price per nutrient, you're getting a bargain. Organic varieties usually don't cost twice as much as the others. The fact that you have to pay more today *not* to have poisonous pesticides in your food is an irony of modern life.

Vegetables are a good source of minerals, but the minerals in plants are usually not as available as those in animals, which have already assimilated them and transformed them into bioavailable forms. One of the best ways to release the minerals from plants is to cook them into soups, simmering them for two or three hours (see next page). The key to getting the most minerals from your vegetables is to retain and drink all the water that they are cooked in, if you boil them, or to stir-fry them without water. Frozen vegetables are usually boiled and drained during processing, stripping away much of the mineral content. See Table 26.12 for a comparison of nutrients in fresh and frozen broccoli.

Mineral and vitamin density varies widely within the fruit and vegetable groups. Unfortunately, the vegetables consumed most often by Americans, such as tomatoes, oranges, bananas, potatoes, and corn, are among the least nutritious of the category. Table 26.13 lists fruits and vegetables in the order of their nutritional value, and compares that order to the most common fruits and vegetables consumed by Americans.

TABLE 26.12   NUTRIENTS LOST IN FROZEN
BROCCOLI (PER 100 GRAMS)

Nutrient	Fresh	Frozen	% Change
Calcium	48 mg	51 mg	+6.25
Phosphorus	66 mg	55 mg	–16.67
Iron	0.88 mg	0.61 mg	–30.68
Potassium	325 mg	180 mg	–44.62
Magnesium	25 mg	20 mg	–20.00
Vitamin A	1,542 IU	1,892 IU	+22.70
Thiamine	0.065 mg	0.055 mg	–15.38
Riboflavin	0.119 mg	0.081 mg	–31.93
Niacin	0.638 mg	0.458 mg	–28.21
Vitamin C	93.2 mg	40 mg	–57.08

Soups

We saw in Chapter 25 that canned soup is one of the leading sources of calories in the United States and one of the top
ten best-selling items in supermarkets. Table 2.5 shows some
of the nutrients lost in the processing of canned foods. Cooking
vegetables in homemade soups breaks up cell walls and releases
minerals that are not available in raw or lightly cooked vegetables. You can supercharge the mineral nutrition of a homemade
soup by adding kelp, blackstrap molasses (a good substitute for
the hidden sugar in canned soup), and soup bones. Crack the
soup bones and scoop the marrow directly into the soup to get
all the minerals that feed the growing cells of the immune system. If you are curious, eat the marrow raw, the way the Indians
in northern Canada do. It is tasty and slightly sweet. Table 26.14
compares the minerals in canned versus homemade soups and
shows how the addition of a handful of kelp and a spoonful of
blackstrap molasses boosts the mineral nutrition.

TABLE 26.13   NUTRIENT DENSITY VS.
CONSUMPTION OF COMMON
FRUITS AND VEGETABLES

Nutrient Concentration		Frequency of Consumption in a Typical American Diet	
Food	*Rank*	*Food*	*Rank*
Broccoli	1	Tomatoes	1
Spinach	2	Oranges	2
Brussels sprouts	3	Potatoes	3
Lima beans	4	Lettuce	4
Peas	5	Sweet corn	5
Asparagus	6	Bananas	6
Artichokes	7	Carrots	7
Cauliflower	8	Cabbage	8
Sweet potatoes	9	Onions	9
Carrots	10	Sweet potatoes	10
Sweet corn	12	Peas	15
Potatoes	14	Spinach	18
Cabbage	15	Broccoli	21
Tomatoes	16	Lima beans	23
Bananas	18	Asparagus	25
Lettuce	26	Cauliflower	30
Onions	31	Brussels Sprouts	34
Oranges	33	Artichokes	36

Pickles and Sauerkraut

Traditional people in both Europe and Asia have pickled their vegetables since the dawn of recorded history. Pickling, which is fermentation with lactic acid–producing bacteria, has benefits similar to those of milk fermentation. The bacteria predigest the plant constituents, freeing up minerals. The sour lactic acid also has health benefits of its own, helping to regulate the normal bacteria in the gut. For some excellent traditional

TABLE 26.14   MINERALS IN 16 OUNCES
OF CANNED VS. HOMEMADE
VEGETABLE SOUP

	Canned*	Homemade**	Kelp and Molasses Added***
Calcium (mg)	9	15	86
Iron (mg)	0.45	0.89	1
Magnesium (mg)	3	24	51
Potassium (mg)	87	571	1152
Zinc (mg)	0.19	0.35	0.76
Copper (mg)	0.05	0.22	0.44
Manganese (mg)	0.19	0.85	1.71

*Canned vegetarian vegetable in equal proportion to water

**Two medium potatoes, tomatoes, and carrots simmered in two quarts of water

***With 5 grams of kelp and 1 tablespoon of blackstrap molasses added

recipes for making pickles and sauerkraut, see the cookbook *Nourishing Traditions* by Sally Fallon (1995).

The Vegetable Fast

Fasting is a time-honored method for improving the health. For most Americans, whose diet and constitution today is very different from that of traditional people or robust peasant farmers, any kind of prolonged fast does more harm than good. Rather than a strict fast, I recommend a three-day vegetable fast for many of my clients. Eat only vegetables—as many as you want, in whatever form you want—for three days. This helps to cleanse the digestive tract and gives the system a rest from digesting fats and proteins, but it also helps to remineralize a run-down body.

Juicing

We saw in Chapter 3 that some of our fruits and vegetables have lost much of their mineral content during the last eighty years. Figure 3.1 shows that certain plants today contain only about one-fifth of the minerals they contained in 1914. You may be able to push that to one-third by buying organic vegetables, which contain on average about twice the minerals as commercial produce. You can get all the minerals back by making fresh juices with organic fruits and vegetables. If you juice three organic carrots, apples, and celery stalks, and have them for a morning drink, you'll be getting most of the minerals that your ancestors did in 1914 when they ate one apple, carrot, and piece of celery.

I recommend a glass of fresh-squeezed juice four or five days a week, or even daily if you tolerate it well. I don't recommend overdoing juices, or going on prolonged juice fasts, because juices are very cooling to the system and can impair digestion. If you find even a single glass of vegetable juices too cooling, try juicing a clove of garlic along with the other items. Large amounts of fruit juices contain large amounts of fruit sugar, which, like refined sugar, can depress the immune system. Let vegetables make up the largest portion of your fresh-squeezed juice. For excellent information on juicing, see *The Complete Book of Juicing* by Michael Murray, N.D. (1992).

SALT

Animals will travel miles to a salt lick, and humans have gathered salt from seashores or ancient seabeds and traded it since the dawn of civilization. Salt was traded during the Middle Ages with a value about the same as gold. The salt that animals eat at salt licks and that traded by our ancestors differ greatly in mineral content from the salt you buy in supermarkets today.

TABLE 26.15   MINERALS IN SALT (PARTS PER MILLION)

Mineral	Sea Salt	Table Salt
Chloride	490,000	612,262
Sodium	310,000	387,400
Sulfur	11,200	0
Zinc	9,200	0.01
Magnesium	7,200	10.1
Iron	3,800	3.4
Potassium	2,900	80.8
Manganese	2,600	0.01
Calcium	2,200	242.5
Copper	1,800	0.003
Silicon	1,100	0
Strontium	90	0
Boron	80	0
Fluorine	40	0
Lithium	2	0
Rubidium	1.4	0
Phosphorus	1.12	0
Iodine	0.7	0
		(unless iodized)
Barium	0.2	0
Molybdenum	0.12	0
Nickel	0.8	0
Arsenic	0.037	0
Manganese	0.024	0
Vanadium	0.024	0
Tin	0.009	0
Cobalt	0.004	0
Antimony	0.003	0
Silver	0.003	0
Chromium	0.002	0
Mercury	0.002	0
Cadmium	0.001	0
Selenium	0.001	0

Note: Sea salt contains the other mineral elements of the sea at levels of parts per billion or parts per trillion, which are insignificant to humans

Table 26.15 shows the comparison between the minerals in table salt and sea salt. Table salt is almost pure sodium chloride, whereas sea salt contains about 20 percent of other minerals and trace elements by weight. I will also describe some seawater concentrates in Chapter 29 that may be used as substitutes for salt in cooking.

SEA VEGETABLES

Seaweeds are a treasured food throughout the world wherever traditional people have access to them. Weston Price found a man high in the Andes mountains who was carrying kelp and fish eggs in his pack. The foods had been traded hundreds of miles into the mountains, carried all the way from the sea. Kelp and other seaweeds were used by the Irish as supplemental foods, garden fertilizers, and survival foods during periods of famine. Eskimos are known to go out in the dead of winter storms to break the ice and gather seaweeds.

Table 26.16 shows the mineral content of some seaweeds. Kelp—a common name for seaweeds in several seaweed genuses—is by far the richest in minerals. The kelp *Fucus vesiculosus*, also called bladderwrack, from the North Atlantic has been used as a nutritional supplement and medicine in coastal areas throughout recorded European history. Kelp can vary between 25 and 50 percent minerals by dry weight, and a five-gram daily dose (still containing some moisture) may contain a gram or two of minerals. Most of the trace elements are not in the table, because figures are not available for them, but sea plants in general contain most of the mineral elements of the sea, with some of them highly concentrated from seawater (see Table 1.3). As we saw in Chapter 1, the mineral content of sea plants is close to the same proportion as the mineral content in the nuclei of your cells, evidence of the interconnectedness of

TABLE 26.16   MINERAL CONTENT OF SOME
SEAWEEDS (PER 100 GRAMS)

Nutrient	Kelp	Irish Moss	Wakame
Calcium (mg)	3,040	72	150
Iron (mg)	1.6	8.9	2.18
Magnesium (mg)	867	144	107
Potassium (mg)	2,110	63	50
Zinc (mg)	0.06	1.95	0.38
Copper (mg)	0.13	0.149	0.284
Manganese (mg)	0.76	0.37	1.4
Vitamin A (IU)	6,600	118	360
Folate (mcg)	n/a	182	196

(Sources: *Fucus vesiculosus*, from Pedersen, 1993; U.S. Department of Agriculture, 1997)

all life on the cellular level. Sea plants are, in general, a better source of minerals than sea salt, because the proportions of minerals are closer to those in the human body.

The upside of sea vegetables for Americans in the 1990s is that harvesting sea vegetables cannot deplete the ocean the way farming does to the soil, and they contain the same rich mineral content that our ancestors valued so highly. Because seaweeds grow in coastal waters, and because our civilization uses those waters as a toilet for human and industrial wastes, it is important to get seaweeds from clean areas of the coasts. I list several sources in Appendix B.

A healthy dose of kelp is three to five grams, dried, a day. Kelp contains a large molecular weight carbohydrate called algin, which may bind to the minerals or impair their absorption in the intestine. Algin extracts are sold separately as weight loss products, because they inhibit caloric absorption. It is my opinion that the algin in seaweeds, at three- to five-gram doses, does not effectively inhibit the absorption of minerals. I have seen so many individuals benefit from the addition of kelp to their diet. Individuals who have trouble digesting kelp may put it in soups the way the Japanese do. Larger doses, with more algin, may begin to inhibit the absorption of other foods and cause imbalances. Take seaweeds as they are, roast them lightly, grind them up and use them like salt, or cook them in soups. Don't cook them for more than about 30 minutes, however, because this can release toxic heavy metals from plants harvested from polluted waters (Drum, 1997).

HERBS AND SPICES

Traditional herbal medicines and cooking spices contain large amounts of minerals and trace elements. An ounce of many dried herbs contains far higher mineral content than even three ounces of fruits, vegetables, or other plant foods—sometimes more than ten times the amount. Table 26.17 lists the mineral content of some herbs that are traditionally consumed as beverage teas. To get this kind of mineral content, buy herbs that have been harvested in the wild (or harvest them yourself). Farmed herbs are subject to the same dynamics of soil depletion as other agricultural plants. The best way to get the mineral content from these herbs is to put an ounce each of two or three of them in the bottom of your drip coffeemaker. Add water to the back, and let the herbs simmer on the hot plate for a few hours, stirring occasionally and crushing the plant material from time to time. Many cooking spices, in tablespoon amounts, also contain significant mineral nutrients.

MAKING CHANGES

The dietary changes discussed in this chapter may seem overwhelming, and it may take effort to find some of the foods men-

TABLE 26.17 MINERAL CONTENT OF SELECTED HERBS
(MILLIGRAMS OF MINERAL PER OUNCE OF HERB)

Herb	Calcium	Chromium	Iron	Magnesium	Manganese	Potassium	Selenium	Silicon	Zinc
Alfalfa	299	0.03	0.87	76	0.08	400	0	0	0
Burdock	244	0.01	4.9	179	0.20	560	0.05	0.75	0.07
Catnip	205	0.09	4.6	69	1.25	783	0.41	0	0
Chickweed	403	0.04	8.4	176	0.18	280	0.14	0.19	0.17
Comfrey leaf	600	0.06	0.4	23	0.19	566	0.04	0.30	0
Horsetail	630	0.01	4.1	145	0.23	520	0.04	1.29	0
Kelp	1,013	0.02	0.5	289	0.25	703	0.06	0.03	0.02
Licorice	292	0.06	2.9	321	0.16	380	0	0.53	0.01
Marshmallow	272	0.05	3.8	172	0.15	403	0.11	0.10	0
Nettle Leaf	966	0.13	1.4	286	0.26	583	0.07	0.34	0.16
Oatstraw	476	0.13	0.4	400	0.02	90	0.04	0.61	0
Peppermint	540	0	2.0	220	0.02	753	0.04	0.00	0
Red Clover	436	0.11	0	116	0.20	666	0.03	0.04	0
Red Raspberry	403	0.04	3.3	106	4.80	446	0.08	0.04	0
Skullcap	151	0.02	0.8	37	0.16	726	0.03	0.16	0.29

(Source: Pedersen, 1994)

tioned. Weston Price found that traditional people often went to great lengths to obtain nutritious foods—sometimes walking dozens of miles or breaking ice in a winter storm to get a certain mineral-rich plant. As Americans in the 1990s, we will have to make some effort as well. The foods I recommend here may be more expensive than the ones you are eating now. But the way I see it, they are not any more expensive *per unit of nutritional value* than supermarket foods. An herbalist I know tells her clients, "If you won't spend time getting well, you'll spend time being sick." My corollary to that is, "If you won't invest in your health, you'll first spend time feeling sick, tired, anxious, and depressed; then you'll spend a lot of time and money on your chronic illnesses."

In my experience, dietary changes are most difficult in the first six weeks. Our dietary tastes are habits, they're not inborn. If you invest some extra effort during the first six weeks, your appetite will gradually change, and you'll start looking forward to new, more nutritious foods. The changes I recommend here are almost all delicious foods. Have a ball and enjoy the food. The nutritional urge is one of the most fundamental, and when your body starts feeling nourished, you will feel like jumping up and dancing. I recommend changes in three stages: additions, substitutions, and, finally, eliminations. And you can still eat some "forbidden" foods every week or so, on the occasion of a feast. The sections that follow summarize the recommendations in this chapter.

Step 1 : Additions

More fruits and vegetables, including homemade pickles
   and sauerkraut
Fresh, homemade vegetable juice
Wild fish one or two days a week

Fermented soy products, such as tempeh and miso, one or
   two days a week
Organic organ meats, such as liver, one day a week
Soak your grains overnight before cooking them
Extra-virgin olive oil for stir-frying and salad dressings
Sea vegetables, especially kelp, as a supplementary
   vegetable or condiment
Butter, if you've previously removed it from your diet for
   health reasons
Blackstrap molasses as a condiment and a sweetener for
   cooked foods
Fresh, refrigerated flaxseed oil
Fresh ground organic flax seeds, as a condiment
Herbal teas

Step 2: Substitutions

Fresh vegetables for canned or frozen varieties
Homemade soups for canned varieties
Organic fruits and vegetables for supermarket varieties
Lamb or game meat for other red meats
Wild fish for other meats
Whole grains for processed varieties
Fresh-cracked grains for commercial flours and oatmeal
Porridges from presoaked grains for bread
Whole raw milk for pasteurized lowfat milk
Fermented dairy products, such as yogurt, for milk
Blackstrap molasses for other sweeteners
Olive oil and butter for refined vegetable oils
Fresh homemade vegetable juices or naturally
   sweetened herbal teas for soft drinks and
   sugar-sweetened juices
Sea salt for table salt

Step 3: Eliminations

All forms of sugar, including hidden sugars in soft drinks
and most processed foods
Deep-fried oils
Refined vegetable oils
Margarine and other hydrogenated oils and shortenings
Caffeine, nicotine, and alcohol
Over-the-counter drugs

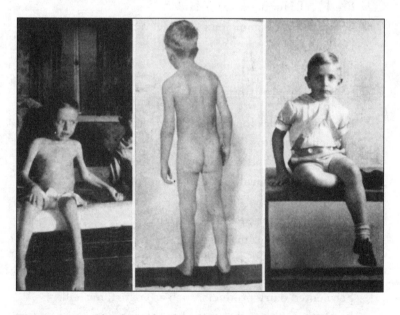

Figure 26.2   This boy, age five, had suffered for two and one-half years from inflammatory rheumatism, arthritis, and heart involvement. Upper left shows limit of movement of neck, left wrist, swollen knees, and ankles. The middle upper view shows the change in six months after improvement of his nutrition, and at right his change in one year. (Photos and caption reprinted from Price, 1938.)

CONCLUSION

I began this chapter asking whether dietary changes can cure disease. I've presented facts through the chapter suggesting that they can. For some graphic evidence, see Figure 26.2. This five-year-old boy had been suffering from arthritis, rheumatic fever with heart involvement, and severe tooth decay. He spent most of his time in bed. Doctors had declared that he would not recover. Weston Price suggested a simple nutritional program that included the elimination of sugar and white flour products, replacing them with fresh-cracked or ground whole wheat. Small amounts of high-vitamin butter (from cows pasturing on green wheat) were added, along with small doses of vitamin-rich cod liver oil. Liver, fresh raw whole milk, and liberal amounts of green vegetables and fruits were included. Bone marrow was added to stews. These were the only changes that could account for the radiant health of the boy after one year. Six years later, his mother reported that he was taller and heavier than average for his age, and that he ate and slept well.

If these simple dietary changes, emphasizing vitamin- and mineral-rich whole foods as they occur in nature, can restore health in such an advanced organic disease as this, it can benefit the many functional diseases that beset us—fatigue, depression, anxiety, immunodepression, and so on. Notice that animal foods, including fat, meat, and butter, were key parts of the program. In the next chapter I will question the long-term therapeutic value of both lowfat and vegetarian diets.

CHAPTER 27

THERAPEUTIC DIETS

Several diets in the United States—lowfat, vegetarian, and macrobiotic—have reputations as "healthy" diets. Although the short-term benefits of these diets are well-documented, people who follow them for too long may develop mineral and other deficiencies.

I was fortunate enough in 1979 to meet Dr. Paavo Airola, a naturopath and a popular writer on nutrition in the 1970s and 1980s, before he died. He explained something at the time that clarified many of my questions about diet, and which has stayed with me ever since. He said, "You have to understand the difference between a therapeutic diet and a sustaining diet." A therapeutic diet can help cure disease, especially the Western diseases. After a time, however, it may cease to sustain health and begin to cause deficiency syndromes. Many adherents to therapeutic diets initially obtain tremendous health benefits, some even apparently miraculous. They then become almost religiously attached to the diet. If they become too dogmatic, when new deficiencies begin to set in they will deny that it is due to the diet, and fail to make a transition to a healthy sustaining diet. The modified sustaining diet usually can retain most of the beneficial elements of the therapeutic diet but requires the reintroduction of foods formerly thought of as "forbidden."

In this chapter, I'll describe three types of diets that are excellent therapeutic diets, but which may cause problems if adhered to dogmatically for a long time.

LOWFAT DIETS

The contemporary therapeutic diet with the most scientific validation is undoubtedly the lowfat diet, urged today to prevent heart disease and some forms of cancer. The Ornish and Pritikin Diet plans, both of which can reverse serious atherosclerosis, employ a radically lowfat diet (less than 10 percent fat), increase fruits and vegetables, exclude sugar and processed foods, and encourage exercise. The fat content of these diets is modeled after that in Japan and many third world countries where levels of heart disease, cancer, and other Western diseases are low.

The problem with multiple dietary changes like this is that the results cannot be attributed to any one of the factors. The benefits may be due entirely to the exclusion of sugar and processed food and the increased fruits, vegetables, and exercise, and have nothing to do with the decreased fat. China and Japan have lowfat diets and low incidence of degenerative disease, but so does France, where people consume a high-fat diet (see Tables 27.1 and 27.2). The Chinese and Japanese also have low consumption of sugars and processed foods, which could account for the lower disease rates as well. People in some areas of the Mediterranean consume 30 percent fat in their diets—mostly from fish and olive oil—and also have low rates of heart disease and cancer. Weston Price found that many traditional peoples consumed about 35 percent fat in their diets—all of it from animals—yet remained free of Western

TABLE 27.1   HEART ATTACKS PER
100,000 PEOPLE

Country	Rate	Fat in the Diet
Japan	34	Low fat, high fish consumption
France	58.6	High fat, high butter consumption
Italy	94.7	High fat, high olive oil consumption
United States	170	High fat, low fish, butter, and olive oil consumption

(Source: U.S. Department of Commerce, 1996)

disease. Other epidemiological evidence suggests that animal fat, in the context of a traditional diet low in processed foods, is actually healthier than fat from oil sources:

• A study compared the health of Jews living in Yemen, who consumed only animal fats and no sugar, to that of Jews in Israel, whose diets include vegetable oils and margarine and 25 percent caloric intake from sugar. The Yemeni Jews had little heart disease, but those in Israel had high levels, as well as more diabetes (Cohen, 1963).

• A similar trial compared groups in northern and southern India. Those in northern India, who consume seventeen times more animal fat, had only one-seventh the risk of heart disease (Malhotra, 1968).

The lowfat dietary dogma also ignores inconsistencies in many contemporary scientific trials. For instance:

• The Framingham Heart Study, initiated in 1948, investigated the diets of about six thousand people in the town of Framingham, Massachusetts. The health of a group consuming little cholesterol and saturated fat was compared, at five year intervals, with a group that consumed more. This study is often cited as proof of the link between high blood cholesterol and

TABLE 27.2   LIFE EXPECTANCY AND
FAT CONSUMPTION

Country	Average Life Expectancy (Years)	Fat in the Diet
Japan	79.6	Low fat, high fish consumption
Austria	79.4	High fat
Canada	79.1	High fat
France	78.4	High fat, high butter consumption
Greece	78.1	High fat, high fish and olive oil consumption
Sweden	78.1	High fat
Italy	78.0	High fat, high olive oil consumption
United States	76.0	High fat

(Source: U.S. Department of Commerce, 1996)

the risk of heart attacks. What most commentators do not mention however, is that the heart attack risk is *inversely* correlated with consumption of cholesterol and saturated fat. The current director of the study writes: "In Framingham, Mass., the more saturated fat one ate, the more cholesterol one ate, the more calories one ate, the lower the person's serum cholesterol. . . . We found that the people who ate the most cholesterol, ate the most saturated fat, and ate the most calories, weighed the least and were the most physically active (Castelli, 1992)."

• A trial in Britain compared the health of a group of men who reduced saturated fat and cholesterol in their diets, quit smoking, and increased their intake of margarine and vegetable oils with another group who did not make these changes. After twelve months, twice as many men on the lowfat, "good" diet had died, even though the other men continued to smoke (Rose, 1983).

• The U.S. Multiple Risk Factor Intervention Trial compared the diet and mortality rate of more than twelve thousand
men. Those who smoked less and consumed less saturated fat
and cholesterol had a slight reduction in heart attacks, but their
overall mortality from all causes was higher (*Journal of the American Medical Association*, 1982).

• More than half of all patients with atherosclerosis do
not have any of the conventional risk factors such as diabetes,
high blood pressure, high cholesterol, obesity, or smoking
(Constantini et al., 1997).

Despite some inconsistencies like these, a positive correlation between total fat and animal fat probably does exist in
Western societies. But that correlation does not exist in a vac-
uum. Low exercise, low consumption of fruits and vegetables,
high consumption of sugar and refined foods, high margarine
consumption, and progressive demineralization of the soil and
foods grown from it also exist. We simply don't know, scientifically, which of these factors causes the disease. Lowfat diets and
a reduction of animal fat may make sense if you otherwise con-
tinue to eat the standard American diet. The need to do so may
disappear if you make the kind of dietary changes recommended
in the last chapter and exercise at a reasonable level. Exercise is
not the subject of this book, but thirty to forty-five minutes of
walking a day will cut your risk of heart disease in half, and your
risk of cancer by a third, changes which may greatly outweigh
any risk that comes from consuming animal fat.

One of the strongest risk factors for heart attacks—
stronger than the risk presented by fat in the diet—is sugar
consumption. People consuming more than four ounces of
sugar a day, which is only two-thirds of the per capita average
in the United States, have five times the risk of heart attack of
those who consume two ounces or less (Glinsmann et al., 1986).

Current research indicates that the best predictor of atherosclerosis is not serum cholesterol, but high levels of the protein metabolite homocysteine. Vitamin B_6, vitamin B_{12}, and folic acid, all of which are high in animal products and removed in the processing of whole grains, will lower serum homocysteine levels. The antioxidant mineral selenium is also associated with atherosclerosis, and the antioxidant vitamin E will dramatically reduce risks of a heart attack. The consumption of fat, in the presence of adequate levels of these vitamins and minerals, may have no correlation to atherosclerosis at all.

The long-term effects of lowfat diets on Americans is not known. My chief concerns about them are:

- They may also be low in essential fatty acids.
- They may be low in the fat-soluble vitamins A, D, and E.
- They may be low in minerals and trace elements.
- When people binge on fat or oils while otherwise following a lowfat diet, they may consume large amounts of an unhealthy oil.

The original Pritikin Diet allowed no added fat or oil at all. Compliance with the diet was poor, and those who could stay with it soon developed fatigue, difficulty with concentration, depression, weight gain, and various mineral deficiencies (Gittleman, 1980). Pritikin then modified the diet to include about 10 percent calories from fat. If you are following the Pritikin or Ornish Diets, there is no reason, from the point of cardiovascular health, not to add fish to your diet. Fish has a protective effect on the heart and arteries.

It remains to be seen whether these diets are healthy, sustaining diets. Pritikin died in his early sixties. Proponents of the diet point out that his arteries were free from atherosclerosis, although his coronary arteries had been blocked during his

CASE STUDY #1

I had a client recovering from surgery for breast cancer who was afraid to eat tofu because it is "high fat." The fat in tofu, however, is about 50 percent essential fatty acids and should not be lumped with the deep-fried oils in fast food french fries.

CASE STUDY #2

A forty-six-year-old man began to develop high cholesterol and triglycerides, and consulted a naturopathic physician for advice. He eliminated wheat (an allergen for him) from his diet and ate a completely vegan diet—no meat or dairy products—with no added oil of any sort, for a month. At the end of this time his cholesterol had returned to near normal and his triglycerides had dropped substantially. The doctor discussed publishing the case in a journal as a demonstration of the possible effects of diet on cholesterol in a compliant patient. After another thirty days, the "bad" cholesterol had returned to the normal range, but his triglycerides shot up to four times the high-normal level. The doctor decided that he had genetically high triglycerides.

The man's diet diary showed that he went to a movie theater once or twice a week and ordered unbuttered popcorn. Even unbuttered popcorn contains large amounts of palm kernel oil however, and a dietary analysis showed that he was getting 9 percent of his weekly calories from the two servings of popcorn. The single oil in the diet completely unbalanced his ability to regulate blood lipids. He returned to his normal diet, which was mostly vegetables but included some commercial chicken. The cholesterol remained just above the high-normal level and the triglycerides dropped by half to twice the high-normal levels. A year later, he introduced regular fish and organic-only vegetables to his diet, and all blood lipids returned to normal levels.

forties. Nevertheless, he died of leukemia about a decade earlier than the average life expectancy for men in the United States.

This section is not an invitation to chow down on hamburgers or to ignore your level of obesity. But the demonization of animal fat is inconsistent with known epidemiological evidence from traditional societies who were completely free from the Western diseases now attributed to fat consumption.

Vegetarianism

A vegetarian diet is perhaps the most famous of the "healthy" diets. It is not a natural diet for humans, however. The closest thing to a vegetarian diet that Weston Price found among traditional people was that of the alpine Swiss. They consumed mostly grains and dairy products, but ate meat about once a week. One set of African tribes ate mostly agricultural foods, but they also consumed some meat from cattle and goats, frogs, insects, and insect eggs. The rest of the traditional people studied consumed large amounts of meat, and all groups were free of the most common diseases in the West today.

In our clinic in Boulder, we see a steady stream of sick vegetarians, perhaps 40 percent of our clients. They are usually fatigued, depressed, or anxious, with low-grade inflammatory conditions, frequent colds, and they often try to compensate for these problems by smoking too much marijuana. We have dubbed them the "fast food vegetarians," because, although they refrain from meat, they do *not* refrain from sugar, processed flour and oils, and other mineral-depleting foods, and they don't take the time to cook nutritious meals. A typical breakfast might be a bagel (with white flour and sugar) and cream cheese. No meat, but nothing else nutritious either. As we'll see following, it may be possible for Americans to maintain health on a vegetarian diet, but they have to work at it and be even more careful than meat eaters about eating the "foods of civilization."

I followed a strict vegetarian diet from 1973 until 1986 and was mostly vegetarian for another five years. Before adopting the diet I was quite sickly, and the combination of eating a vegetarian diet, eliminating sugars and refined foods, stopping my addictions, and regular exercise restored me to a level of health I had not thought possible. For the first twelve years, I was so healthy that I did not take so much as an aspirin for medication, and only rarely took mild medicinal herb teas.

Eventually, however, I was so run down I couldn't function at my job and became allergic to many of the foods I ate. My spiritual teacher at the time, who practiced in the Hindu tradition, advised that I should not eat meat until I had asked myself a thousand times whether I could maintain a healthy body without participating in the killing of animals. I asked the question of myself for more than a year, and ultimately concluded that I needed the meat. My health improved afterward.

My experience, which may have been caused by the demineralization of our food supply during those years, is not unique. Most of the people I know who were vegetarians in the 1970s now eat at least some meat. The only long-term vegetarians I know today who appear to be healthy are members of some religious groups who are very careful to avoid sugar and processed foods, who eat only organic fruits and vegetables, and who take the time to cook abundant, hearty, well-rounded meals.

THE ROOTS OF AMERICAN VEGETARIANISM

Vegetarianism as an ideology came to the United States through three main routes: the Seventh-Day Adventist movement of the mid-1800s; the Theosophical movement of the late 1800s, which was strongly influenced by Hinduism; and the German naturopathic movement, which came to America at the turn of the century.

Vegetarians in India

The Hindu religion calls for a vegetarian diet. I will not debate this religious point, and I personally have high regard for the Hindu religion and the many saints it has produced. But I also notice that the different religious traditions revealed in different times and places have different dietary rules. These may be especially important in the regions where they arose. In tropical regions, body-heat regulation is essential, especially when the outside temperature rises above the 98.6-degree temperature of the body. At that point, any kind of heat-generating motion, or even a slight breeze, heats the body rather than cools it as it would in a colder climate. The only available ways to cool the body are to sit still, drink liquids that are cooler than body temperature, consume spices that promote sweating, and reduce the intake of "heating" foods such as meat. It is also difficult to maintain meat in a sanitary condition in hot, tropical climates. Indians also cook and season their food in a way that optimizes absorption of minerals, which are more difficult to assimilate from plants than from animal foods.

I once spent a week in Calcutta in July, where temperatures average about 115 degrees during the day. I was amazed to see how fast the food spoiled there. The scraps of a leftover lunch would be moldy and decayed by late afternoon. I lived almost exclusively on fruits and yogurt during that week because they were the only foods I had an appetite for. For contemplative spiritual purposes, a vegetarian diet calms the mind and cools the passions. Indian yogis traditionally follow a vegetarian diet, which promotes their meditation, but they also spend hours of the day sitting still and do not work in the world, reducing their nutrient requirements.

Indians may also be better adapted genetically to vegetarianism. We saw in the last chapter that the EPA from fish and wild game is the most easily metabolized of the essential fatty acids. Manufacturing EPA from vegetable oil sources (alpha-linolenic acid) within the body requires a complicated pathway involving four enzymes and several vitamins and minerals. It is possible that Indians have developed these pathways efficiently over their many generations of vegetarianism. An active American, descended from fish- and game-eating Europeans, who leads a busy active life in a cold climate, who does not take the time to cook and season the foods as the Indians do, and who eats progressively demineralized American plant foods may not thrive at all on a vegetarian diet.

India as a nation is not exclusively vegetarian, but comes closer to it than any other society. And even in India a vegetarian diet may not be optimum, from a health point of view. The life expectancy in India is less than sixty years. Even adjusted for the high infant mortality rate, it rises only to about sixty-four, more than a decade less than even Americans who eat a poor diet. The vegetarians of southern India have one of the shortest average life spans on earth (Abrams, 1980). Furthermore, even vegetarians in India consume meat in the form of insect and larva contamination of grains. They make a significant enough contribution to the diet that when Indian vegans move to England, where food products have higher standards of cleanliness, they develop higher rates of pernicious anemia, due to a lack of vitamin B_{12}.

Seventh-Day Adventists

Several clinical trials have shown that vegetarian Seventh-Day Adventists are generally healthier than the average American. These studies are sometimes put forward as proof that vegetarianism is a healthy diet. Adventists have lower rates of atherosclerosis and some kinds of cancer. However, these benefits may not come from the absence of meat, but from the absence of sugar and refined foods, and from other foods they *do* eat. Seventh-Day Adventists eat no refined foods but plenty of fruits and vegetables. I tell my clients that if they want to be vegetarian, they should model their diets after the Adventist diet.

The Naturopaths

Although the German naturopaths advised and employed vegetarianism as a therapeutic diet, there was no consensus among them that it is a sustainable diet. Vincent Priessnitz, the founder of the German naturopathic movement, fed his patients high-quality meat and milk to give them strength to endure the cold-water hydrotherapy treatments he administered. J. H. Rausse, a successor to Priessnitz, lived in America for a time among the Osage Indians, hunting and eating wild fish and game. Vegetarianism was only introduced into the naturopathic movement in Germany by Theodore Hahn, fifty years after Priessnitz had launched it. Hahn, who followed this diet for his entire life, died at age fifty-nine. Influential naturopath Arnold Rikli, who practiced nature cure for the last fifty years of the nineteenth century, then promptly rejected the vegetarian diet as a sustainable one. Under Hahn's guidance, Rikli had adopted a vegetarian diet at age thirty-eight. His health thrived for about twelve years, but eventually he developed chronic fatigue, heart palpitations, poor mood, brittle fingernails, and a loss of body heat, all signs of mineral deficiency, and the same set of symptoms I see in long-term vegetarians in our clinic today. After two years of eating a small portion of meat each day, all the symptoms disappeared. He concluded that vegetarianism was excellent as a temporary therapy, but not suitable for everyone as a permanent diet. He also believed that a patient's occupation and constitution must be taken into account when deciding the optimal diet: "A diet which may be right for the blacksmith may not be right for the tailor." Rikli lived to be eighty-three years old, outliving the vegetarian Hahn by thirty-four years.

The succeeding German naturopaths invariably used a vegetarian diet therapeutically, but did not approach it dogmatically, and most fed their patients meat occasionally and ate it at least occasionally themselves. Heinrich Lahmann, who practiced at the end of the nineteenth century, fed his spa patients a large feast once a week:

> *It is certainly good for the neurasthenic [chronic fatigue patient], in fact for everybody, to deviate from his ordinary [healthful] diet once every week or two; I even arrange for this in my sanatorium by giving stimulating dishes every now and then. This is not only harmless, but even useful. The important point is, how we feed ourselves the other six days of the week. (Kirchfeld and Boyle, 1994)*

The great American naturopath Henry Lindlahr, who ran a two hundred–bed inpatient facility in Chicago in the first decades of this century, severely criticized ideological vegetarians for their mental rigidity. He stated that he ate some meat from time to time simply to prevent that sort of thinking from arising in his mind. Lindlahr had a radical turnaround in his health by adopting a vegetarian diet at about age forty. He had been dying of diabetes before that. He maintained this mostly vegetarian diet for another twenty-two years, until he died at age sixty-two of a simple infection, presumably from a deficient immune system.

Vegans

A vegan is a vegetarian who eats no animal products at all, omitting even dairy products and eggs. This is an excellent short-term therapeutic diet, especially for someone deficient in minerals and poisoned by modern foods. The omission of dairy, a common allergen, helps many people to regain their health. But this diet is an even worse sustaining diet than a broader vegetarian diet. The change in my own diet in the mid-1980s that precipitated my general failure of health was eliminating dairy from my already vegetarian diet.

Table 27.3 shows the low level of omega-3 fatty acids in the breast milk of vegan mothers.

Deficiencies in Vegetarians

If Arnold Rikli emphasized that we need to consider constitution and occupation when selecting the diet, we also need to consider time and place. As we saw in Chapter 3, our foods, especially our fruits and vegetables, are rapidly losing their mineral content—perhaps 25 percent of calcium, magnesium, and the trace elements in the last thirty years. Even if strict vegetarian diets still have some short-term therapeutic value for

TABLE 27.3   OMEGA-3 FATTY ACID
COMPOSITION OF
HUMAN BREAST MILK

People	% of Total Fat
Japanese	2.5
American	1.9
Vegan	1.5

the average American today, they are even less sustainable than they were in Germany a hundred years ago. Vitamins and minerals are more poorly absorbed from plant foods than from meats. The vegetarians I see in our clinic today generally have three or four of the functional deficiency syndromes listed in Table 25.1. As therapy, I advise them to remove all sugars and other refined foods from their diet, and start eating only organic fruits and vegetables, high-quality, omega-3-rich fish, and, if they have a taste for red meat, grass-fed organic lamb. Unfortunately, most are unwilling to change their dogmatic attitudes and want a magic-bullet herbal treatment for their problems instead.

THE MACROBIOTIC DIET

The Zen macrobiotic diet was developed by George Ohsawa in the mid-1900s and has been widely promoted in the United States by his student Mishio Kushi ever since. As a movement, macrobiotics has had a strong influence on the awareness of the value of whole natural foods among the American public since the early 1970s. The diet is based on the use of traditional Japanese foods such as rice, soy products, and seaweeds. I classify it as an excellent therapeutic diet for most Americans, but as a sustaining diet, it has severe pitfalls.

The upside of the macrobiotic diet is that it emphasizes whole, organic, unrefined foods along with the consumption of healthy soy products and mineral-rich seaweeds. It thus eliminates virtually all of the "foods of civilization" and provides excellent dietary therapy for many of the Western diseases. The downside is that, although macrobiotics promotes some traditional foods, its proponents are less enthusiastic about one of the most important Japanese food categories: fish and other sea animals. Although macrobiotic adherents are "allowed" to eat some fish, a vegetarian version of the diet is encouraged.

The macrobiotic diet, as promoted in the United States, is no one's traditional diet, but is a recent theoretical invention. The term *macrobiotic* was borrowed from the German Julius Hensel. Ohsawa added a version of the yin and yang theory of Asian philosophy and medicine to Hensel's organic vegetarian dietary model. This version of yin and yang theory differs in some substantial ways from that of traditional Chinese medicine, however. I studied Chinese medicine in a medical school and find the basis for the macrobiotics version of yin and yang incomprehensible. In traditional Chinese medicine, meat-eating is encouraged and is in fact prescribed medicinally. The macrobiotic adherents consider most meat to be too yang, and avoid it.

Mineral and other nutrient deficiencies from long-term macrobiotic diets are well-documented in the scientific literature. The most common deficiencies are of vitamins D and B_{12}, iron, and protein (American Cancer Society, 1989, 1993). The progressive demineralization of our vegetable foods may also mean more serious problems for dogmatic macrobiotic practitioners in the future, although their regular consumption of mineral-rich sea vegetables may prevent this.

CONCLUSION

The apparent benefits of the three diets discussed in this chapter can ultimately be the source of problems for adherents of the diets. After experiencing the initial benefits, practitioners of these diets may develop a kind of religious attachment to the diet. Then, as long-term mineral deficiencies begin to develop, it becomes difficult to make changes. Each of the diets here is composed mainly of plant foods. In the next chapter, I'll briefly discuss factors that affect the assimilation of minerals, including the difficulty of obtaining minerals in a usable form from plants.

CHAPTER 28

ABSORPTION

You're not what you eat, you're what you absorb.

Joe Boucher, N.D.

You can eat a mineral-rich diet and still develop deficiencies! As far as the body is concerned, nutrition happens only at the cellular level. The foods containing the minerals have to be digested; the minerals are transported from the digestive tract to the blood and on to the cells, and then across the cell membranes. In this chapter, I'll discuss the factors that affect the assimilation of minerals.

AVAILABILITY IN FOODS

In Chapter 2, I listed the nutrients present in a large number of foods. Don't expect to take in everything on the list. Table 28.1 shows the percentage of minerals that are absorbed in a typical diet that includes both plant and animal foods. We absorb on average only about half the mineral nutrients we eat. Vegetarians who eat exclusively plant foods have even poorer absorption. For instance, about 35 percent of iron from animal sources is absorbed, but only 2.9 percent is absorbed from plant sources. This is why Table 28.1 shows an average of only 5 to 15 percent for people who mix plant and animal foods—the plant foods pull the average down. Under the section on grains in Chapter 26, I described how phytic acid in plants also inhibits the absorption of some minerals, especially zinc. A progressive zinc deficiency is common in vegetarians as they adhere to the diet over a number of years. The mineral availability in plants can be increased by soaking or fermenting them before consumption.

INTERACTIONS BETWEEN MINERALS

Minerals and vitamins must also be taken in a balanced way for optimal absorption. Chapters 5 to 24 list interactions between

TABLE 28.1   NET ABSORPTION OF MINERALS IN NORMAL ADULTS ON DIETS CONTAINING BOTH PLANT AND ANIMAL FOODS

Mineral	Percent Absorption
Calcium	5–40
Chlorine	>95
Chromium	1–3
Cobalt	>50
Copper	25
Fluorine	80–90
Iodine	>50
Iron	5–15
Magnesium	25–50
Manganese	<5
Molybdenum	40–50
Phosphorus	50–60
Potassium	80–90
Selenium	>50
Sodium	>95
Zinc	33

(Source: Braunwald et al., 1987)

some of the minerals and vitamins. Figure 28.1 diagrams the interactions between just the minerals. Mineral deficiencies and mineral excesses can inhibit the absorption or metabolism of a number of other minerals. All the minerals in the diagram affect or are affected by at least one other mineral, and phosphorus interacts with at least ten of them. If we added more of the trace

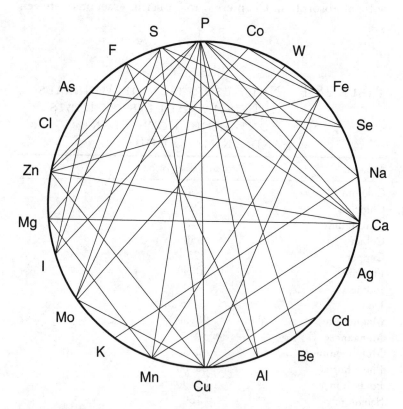

Figure 28.1   Interactions between minerals. Lines indicate that one mineral alters the absorption, metabolism, or excretion of the other. (Source: Ensminger et al., 1983)

elements to the chart, including those that are not yet proven to be essential, the interactions would be even more complex.

The minerals act together like the musicians in a symphony orchestra. If a few key musicians don't show up, the whole orchestra falls apart. And if a few of them start playing too loudly, hogging the show, the others put down their instruments and quit. These complex interactions can be seen in the pathology of the deficiency disease pellagra:

1. Vitamin B_3 becomes deficient.
2. Vitamin B_2, B_6, and the amino acid tryptophan are also likely to be deficient.
3. The B_3 deficiency impairs the absorption of vitamin C.
4. The vitamin C deficiency impairs the absorption of iron.
5. The iron deficiency causes excess absorption of copper.
6. The copper excess inhibits nickel metabolism.
7. The poor nickel metabolism further inhibits iron absorption.

These complex interactions are the best argument to get your minerals from a well-balanced diet containing a wide variety of naturally occurring plant and animal foods. They also argue against relying on supplements of single minerals, a topic I will cover in Chapter 29.

According to the U.S. Department of Agriculture, adult men and women in the United States are on average deficient in both magnesium and zinc (U.S. Department of Agriculture, 1997b). From the diagram, we see that these deficiencies alter the absorption or metabolism of sulfur, phosphorus, iron, calcium, copper, and manganese. Women are also deficient in calcium and iron, which adds cobalt and fluoride to the list. Thus, the average American adult is walking around with disrupted mineral metabolism because of several common deficiencies.

DIGESTION

Poor digestion also can affect absorption. Some signs of poor digestion are:

- Flatulence or belching
- Nausea
- Pain anywhere in the digestive tract
- Undigested food in the stool
- Offensive breath
- Constipation (less than one bowel movement per day)
- Lethargy or depression after meals
- Food cravings other than normal hunger
- Lack of satisfaction after meals
- Lack of hunger for breakfast

If you have any of these symptoms chronically, I'd suggest you get a medical checkup, preferably by a naturopathic or other holistic physician. Some referral sources are listed in Appendix A. If they are minor symptoms that do not accompany any specific disease, I suggest you take the following formula of Western herbs for three to six weeks and see if your overall health and energy improve.

Measure out equal parts of chamomile, peppermint, fennel seed, licorice root, and burdock root. Put a handful of each in a pot and add two quarts of water. Simmer over low heat, with a lid on the pot, for a half hour. Strain and store for future use in a thermos if you have one. Let this be your beverage and drink at least three cups a day. A handy way to make this, if you have a drip coffeemaker, is to put the herbs in the pot (not the strainer) and add water in the back of the coffee maker. Turn it on. The hot water then flows onto the herbs, and the hot plate keeps the herbs at a good simmering temperature without boiling them. You can heat the tea this way for about an hour (less is fine). Strain and store in a thermos to take to work. You can also steep the used herbs again one time, as there will still be plenty of potency left after one brewing. It's important to make enough of this in advance so you don't have to hassle with brewing the tea each time you want a cup. I have often seen seriously run-down clients regain their health within a month using this or similar formulas. The reason is probably the improved absorption of food and the restoration of mineral nutrition to the cells.

Perhaps the most widespread cause of indigestion in the United States today is the habit of eating in stressful or hurried situations. Stress inhibits the secretions of stomach acid and other enzymes that are necessary to digest foods and release their mineral content. I know a naturopathic physician who once cured a woman of her stomach ulcers without any dietary changes, herbs, drugs, enzymes, or any other physical treatment. He simply had her sit relaxed in a chair in a dark room, close her eyes, and mentally recite her favorite prayer for fifteen minutes before her evening meal. The resulting relaxation properly prepared her system for the digestion of food, and the ulcers went away.

Low stomach acid—caused by eating under stress or aging—can impair the absorption of at least eight of the minerals (see Box 28.1). Many people over age sixty produce low stomach acid, or even none at all. The resulting lack of mineral absorption contributes to the aging process. If you think you have low stomach acid, consult a naturopathic or other holistic physician. Acid supplements are available in some health food stores, but I do not consider them appropriate for self-medication.

Herbs that may promote relaxation *and* the secretion of stomach acid and other digestive enzymes are in a class called *bitter nervines*, and include chamomile, skullcap, valerian, and wild yam. These herbs will relax you to varying degrees, and their bitter flavor will promote increased flow of digestive secretions. Take them as warm teas a half hour before mealtime.

BOX 28.1

MINERALS THAT REQUIRE ADEQUATE
STOMACH ACID FOR ABSORPTION

Chromium	Manganese
Copper	Molybdenum
Iron	Selenium
Magnesium	Zinc

(Source: Schauss, 1996)

Chamomile and skullcap are also rich in minerals. If any of these herbs increase your digestive pain, stop taking them right away.

Another category of herbs with a stronger bitter flavor are the *digestive bitters*. These include herbs such as dandelion root, yellow dock, or gentian, in increasing order of bitterness. Gentian preparations have been used as digestive bitters at least since the time of the Greeks. Take digestive bitters if you have poor digestion, flatulence, and a dry tongue (which probably means your stomach is "dry," too). These may be more effective if taken as alcohol preparations twenty minutes before meals. If you have digestive pain, don't take these stronger bitters, because it can increase the pain. You don't need a large dose. Anywhere from three to ten drops is sufficient. The bitter taste on the tongue triggers the digestive secretions.

ABSORPTION

There is no guarantee that minerals, once extracted from digested food, will ever reach the cells in your body. *Malabsorption syndrome* is a recognized problem both in the Western and third world countries. It often accompanies general mineral and vitamin malnutrition because you need some of the nutrients in order to absorb others. Taking large amounts of single vitamin or mineral supplements can also cause this problem. Over-the-counter and prescription drugs can cause digestive malabsorption by disrupting the normal balance of the intestinal bacteria, promoting the overgrowth of yeast in the digestive tract, or injuring the gut wall.

CONCLUSION

We should eat a well-balanced diet with a wide variety of mineral-rich foods. If we take mineral supplements, we should take multivitamins and minerals rather than doses of single nutrients. In the next chapter, I'll discuss supplementation in more detail.

MINERAL
SUPPLEMENTS

As the mineral content of our soil has declined, the general consumption of processed foods has increased, scientists have uncovered widespread mineral and vitamin deficiencies in the population, and the health foods business has boomed. Twenty-five years ago I helped found the first food cooperative in Louisville, Kentucky, so my friends and I could buy brown rice and other whole grains. These items were not for sale anywhere else in town. You can now buy brown rice in any large grocery in the United States.

In the early 1980s I helped introduce the first organic produce for sale in New Haven, Connecticut, at a natural foods grocery I managed. We did more than 40 percent of our business in produce, but due to poor availability, not more than 2 to 3 percent of that was organic. In Boulder, Colorado, where I live now, two stores larger than the one I managed in Connecticut have full produce departments stocked with a majority of organic produce. A local Safeway store even has a larger organic produce section than the New Haven store did. We did only about 5 percent of our business in supplements in the 1980s, although for some other stores, the figure was more than

90 percent. This was a conscious decision, because we felt that eating fresh produce and whole grains, nuts, seeds, cheeses, and other dairy products was healthier than taking supplements. I still feel the same way. In this chapter, I'll discuss mineral supplements, the wisest way to use them, and compare some different forms.

Balance Is Important

Considering the progressive demineralization of our soil and food in the last several generations, it seems reasonable to supplement minerals in your diet. My most adamant advice, however, is to take supplements in a balanced way. Review Figure 28.1 and notice the complex interactions between minerals. If you take calcium alone, it will affect the absorption or metabolism of phosphorus, sulfur, iron, zinc, magnesium, and manganese. These in turn will affect, directly or indirectly, every mineral on the chart! The best way to take them all in their natural proportions is to get them in food, especially from sea plants and animals, grass-fed meats, wild game, and wild herbs. The plant and animal worlds have concentrated minerals in the proportions necessary to sustain life.

But if you want to supplement minerals, use a multi-mineral supplement rather than supplementing with individual minerals. As I described in Chapter 25, it is impossible to develop a deficiency of a single mineral. Like boats in the same harbor, they all fall when the tide goes out, that is, when we consume a mineral-poor diet. Taking one or a few minerals is the equivalent of using NPK fertilizer—which contains only two or three minerals—on burned-out farmland begging for the whole array of trace elements.

A physician of natural medicine might recommend one or several individual mineral supplements for a short time to correct an imbalance. If supplementation continues for too long, however, imbalances will result. I strongly discourage self-medication with single minerals. It is best to take your multi-minerals or trace element supplements in the context of a healthy diet because supplements—no matter how fancy or expensive—are not well-absorbed in the presence of general mineral malnutrition. Supplements are the ultimate fast food, and like other fast food, will not nourish by themselves.

POTENTIAL HARMFUL EFFECTS

Some vitamins may be taken safely in amounts much larger than their recommended dietary allowances. This is not the case with minerals. Many minerals have a toxic range very close to the therapeutic range. For instance, calcium may be taken safely at a dose of about one gram a day. Two grams can disrupt the functions of the parathyroid gland, which regulates calcium metabolism. An herbalist colleague once treated a man for kidney stones. His medical doctors had been unable to determine the ailment's cause, but the herbalist ascertained that the patient was taking large doses of vitamin C to support his heavy athletic workouts. The form of vitamin C he was taking, called Ester-C, also contains calcium; the patient was inadvertently consuming 2.5 grams of calcium a day. The removal of the supplement and addition of some simple herbal treatments resolved the kidney stones (Cabrera, 1993). Box 29.1 shows some of the dangers of supplementing individual minerals at doses higher than their recommended doses. Additional undocumented dangers may exist because doctors do not routinely ask sick patients what vitamin and mineral supplements they are taking, and they do not report adverse effects in the scientific literature.

Supplement Forms

Most minerals today come in one of four forms: mineral salts, chelates, ionic minerals, or colloidal minerals. I'll describe each of these in detail.

Mineral Salts

Most commonly found in supermarkets and drug stores, mineral salts are the least expensive of the forms. They are also more difficult to assimilate than the other forms, and the most likely to cause side effects, such as nausea. They are especially poorly absorbed when the stomach acid is low or other digestive secretions are deficient.

Chelated Minerals

A chelated mineral is attached to an organic molecule, such as a protein. Chelation—from the Greek word for claw—refers to the way the larger molecule grips the mineral. Many minerals occur this way in nature, and hundreds of scientific studies of both humans and animals demonstrate that they are better absorbed than mineral salts. Chelation does not automatically confer better absorption, however. The absorption may depend on the nature of the organic molecule and the requirement of the body for a particular form of a certain mineral. Chromium, copper, iron, magnesium, molybdenum, selenium, and zinc may be best absorbed in their ionic form (Schauss, 1996). A chelate will have to be digested and its mineral released from the organic molecule for maximum absorption. Most of the minerals in high-quality multiple supplements are chelated. I generally recommend using a high-quality multiple vitamin and mineral supplement with the minerals in the form of chelates.

Box 29.1
Some Dangers of Mineral Supplementation

Calcium: Calcium supplementation usually causes no adverse effects at customary doses. Regular doses of more than two grams a day can cause hyperparathyroidism (Shaker et al., 1986). Too much calcium intake relative to phosphorus intake (in a calcium-to-phosphorus ratio greater than 2:1) results in reduced bone strength and interferes with vitamin K metabolism.

Copper: Supplementation should be approached with caution. Elevated levels, sometimes due to contaminated drinking water, can cause profound mental and physical fatigue, poor memory, depression, and insomnia (Nolan, 1983).

Fluoride: Supplementation, even at therapeutic levels, may damage the lining of the stomach (Spak et al., 1989). Fluoride may also increase the risk of bone cancer (National Center for Toxicological Research, 1991).

Germanium: High doses, inorganic impurities in "organic" germanium, and long-term supplementation may be toxic to the kidneys (Schauss, 1991, and Matsusaka et al., 1988). See Chapter 11 for more information.

Iron: The most common side effects of iron supplementation are nausea, vomiting, and stomach pain. Recent research indicates that iron should be supplemented only if it is deficient because an overload in the tissues may cause a wide variety of conditions ranging from frequent infection to cancer (Gordeuk et al., 1987; Halliday and Powell, 1982; and Weinberg, 1984). See Chapter 14 for more information.

(continues)

BOX 29.1

(continued)

Manganese: Chronic manganese toxicity may cause irreversible movement and neurological disorders (Donaldson and Barbeau, 1985). Supplementation may also cause high blood pressure or hypertensive headaches (Pfeiffer and LaMola, 1983).

Selenium: Toxicity from overdose may be associated with hair loss, brittle fingernails, muscular discomfort, skin irritation, nausea, fatigue, immunosuppression, and a garlic odor on the breath (Werbach, 1993).

Zinc: Doses of 100 to 300 milligrams a day for several weeks can impair immunity (Chandra, 1984).

Ionized Minerals

The minerals in seawater occur in an ionized form, like salt dissolved in water. Both the chelates and the ionized minerals are my favorite forms for mineral supplementation. Ionized minerals do not require stomach acid for absorption because they are neither bound together into salts that require dissolution nor bound to organic molecules that require digestion. They are ready, as is, for transport across the gut wall, according to the body's needs. They are especially useful for elders and for people with impaired digestion.

The simplest way to supplement with ionized minerals is to put some sea salt in your soup. The salt dissolves in the soup (not in your stomach acid) and is present there in ionic form. Several companies (see Appendix B) make concentrated seawater supplements that can also be added to soups, breads, or juices. They are naturally high in sodium, so you don't want to overdo them, but they also contain all the minerals of the sea in at least minute concentrations. I have observed dramatic turnarounds in health in some patients after the simple addition of these seawater supplements to the foods in their diet. In addition, I also recommend the addition to the diet of three to five grams a day of kelp. Kelp, like other sea plants, concentrates some minerals to many times the level they occur in seawater (see Table 1.5).

Colloidal Minerals

Colloidal minerals are a new arrival in the mineral marketplace, fueled by a popular sales audiotape distributed by multilevel marketing companies. Colloids are tiny clumps of mineral particles suspended in a liquid. Milk is a familiar example of a colloid, with the particles suspended throughout the water base to make a uniform fluid. Colloidal minerals are controversial, and, in my opinion, a health hazard.

Promoters of these minerals make two major claims: First, that colloidal mineral products contain more than seventy minerals and trace elements, and, second, that they are more readily absorbed than other forms. Neither claim can stand up to the facts. Table 29.1 shows an independent analysis of five leading brands of colloidal minerals, commissioned by Alexander Schauss, Ph.D. The table lists all minerals detected at the level of parts per million. The colloidal companies claim that many other minerals are present at the level of parts per billion or parts per trillion. According to Schauss, modern analytical equipment cannot accurately detect minerals at those levels. A part per million is the equivalent of about a pinch of salt in thirty-two gallons of water. A part per billion would be that same pinch in thirty-two *thousand* gallons of water. That would be thirty-two *million* gallons for a part per trillion. Accurate measurement at such levels is impossible because of background contamination. A single dust particle falling into a test tube would easily yield parts per billion of contamination.

Of the five brands in the table, two contain parts per million of twenty-four minerals, one contains twelve, and two contain only eight. The two with the highest number of minerals also contain toxic minerals, including high amounts of aluminum, discussed later in this chapter. Recommended dietary allowances for trace elements other than iron are not present in a one-ounce dose of any of the colloid supplements. I suspect that the benefits claimed in testimonials of users of these products result from supplementation of iron, which many Americans, especially women, are deficient in. The majority of these products are essentially aluminum supplements, with some iron and insignificant quantities of a few other of the essential minerals and trace elements. To get parts per billion or parts per trillion of the other elements, I urge using sea salt or seawater supplements instead.

Product literature for the companies claims that their minerals are better absorbed than other forms. I performed a thorough search of the MEDLINE computer database of the National Library of Medicine in Bethesda, Maryland, which catalogs scientific articles as far back as 1966. Many absorption studies appear for other forms of minerals, but I could not find a single trial, using either animals or humans as subjects, that analyzed the absorbability of colloidal minerals. Database searching can sometimes miss topics, but two other researchers have done the same investigation and come up with the same results (Binder, 1996, and Schauss, 1996). The best argument against the necessity of taking minerals in the colloidal form comes from

TABLE 29.1   MINERALS PRESENT IN FIVE COMMERCIAL SAMPLES OF
COLLOIDAL MINERALS (CONTENT IN PARTS PER MILLION)*

Essential Minerals	Brand A	B	C	D	E	RDA**
Calcium	0	505	1,180	488	517.6	28,070
Lithium	0.218	5.564	0	0	5.7	n/a
Magnesium	0	500	245	402	694.6	10,526
Potassium	97.4	13	339	0	26.4	70,175
Sodium	22,995.8	81	328	55.3	218.8	17,543
Beryllium	0	0.368	0	0	0	n/a
Boron	18.8	2.31	0	0	8.5	52
Bromide	0	0	0	0	3.4	n/a
Chromium	0	0.841	0	0	0.0132	4,385
Cobalt	0	4.167	0	0	2.1	n/a
Copper	1.3	2.71	0	2.63	0.554	79
Iodine	0	0	0	0	0.006	5.3
Iron	1.3	958.2	330	329	50.3	350
Manganese	0	12.42	0	0	20.1	122

Molybdenum	0	1.921	0	0	1.3	5.6
Nickel	0	9.044	0	0	2.6	n/a
Phosphorus	9.7	0	0	0	10.5	28,070
Silicon	146.9	23.8	42.2	26.2	2.8	n/a
Strontium	0.2	1.011	0	0	78,297.8	n/a
Sulphur	98.1	5,908	0	0	0	n/a
Tin	0.002	0	0	0	0.09	n/a
Vanadium	0	1.232	0	0	0.602	n/a
Zinc	0	32.81	3.8	27.4	13.7	421
Zirconium	0	0.18	0	0	0	n/a
Totals	11	20	7	7	21	

Toxic Minerals

Aluminum	18.2	2,741	338	2,290	4,339.4	n/a
Arsenic	0	1.18	0	0	2.2	n/a
Cadmium	0	0.71	0	0	0	n/a
Lead	0	0.955	0	0	0.006	n/a

*Other elements may be present at the level of parts per billion or parts per trillion. Modern analytical equipment cannot measure accurately at these levels, and they are clinically irrelevant to living organisms (Schauss, 1996)

**Per 1 ounce of colloidal minerals

one company's multilevel marketing tape itself. The lecturer cites many clinical trials to prove that mineral supplementation will cure or prevent many diseases. The vast majority of studies he mentions used mineral salts or chelates, not colloidal minerals.

Most colloidal minerals are made from clay deposits, which naturally contain high amounts of aluminum silicate. This explains the high levels of aluminum in the products. Clay is of interest in medicine, both human and veterinary, because it can bind to poisons in the gut and is sometimes used as an antidote for accidental poisoning (Schell et al., 1993; Unsworth et al., 1989; and Merideth and Vale, 1987). In fact, it binds toxins so effectively that, if given along with some pharmaceutical drugs, it greatly reduces their availability (Thoma and Lieb, 1983). Using clay applications externally and taking small amounts of clay orally are ancient traditions in European natural medicine. I've used clay preparations externally with great success for more than twenty years in my herbal practice. They are useful for some skin irritations, such as poison ivy or oak, and for poisonous insect bites, boils, splinters, infections, and other skin problems. Externally, clay is such a powerful drawing agent that it will extract not only poisons, but even objects like splinters from wounds. Colloidal minerals, however, which have most of the elements in the clay removed, do not have these properties.

The internal use of clay—a naturopathic tradition from Europe—has raised questions about potential aluminum toxicity with long-term use. The physician literature produced by one analytical laboratory that specializes in tissue mineral levels lists the internal use of clay as a leading cause of aluminum accumulation on the body (ARL, 1997). The body normally will absorb only the small amount of aluminum it needs from the intestine. That aluminum is then excreted by the kidneys. If there is any compromise of the gut wall integrity, as may occur in ulcerative conditions or intestinal yeast infections, more aluminum can sneak into the system. If kidney function is impaired, toxic aluminum levels can build up in the body, resulting in toxicity to the nerves. Scientists investigating the possibility that clay products cause this reaction found that aluminum in clay suspensions is not only toxic to the nerves, but it can damage the blood/brain barrier, literally breaking its way into the brain to do its damage. Dementia from aluminum poisoning is widely recognized in medicine, and the experiments show that aluminum in clay can cause this problem (Murphy et al., 1993a and 1993b). The experiments were done in test tubes rather than on human subjects, for obvious reasons. Patients with kidney disease are routinely warned against taking aluminum-containing antacids and they should also avoid the internal use of clay or colloidal minerals. Unfortunately, many cases of kidney disease remain "silent" and undiagnosed until they reach emergency proportions.

Conclusion

Mineral supplements may have their place in our diets, but I strongly recommend that you do not use them as "fast-food" replacement for an otherwise healthy diet. Mineral-rich foods, such as seaweeds, blackstrap molasses, and herbs harvested in the wild, contain their minerals in natural and easily assimilated forms in the balance and proportions we need. The addition of a balanced diet of the natural foods, as discussed in Chapter 26, will provide all the minerals you need (for individuals with impaired digestion, ionic mineral supplements may be necessary).

Spiritual Considerations

Traditional peoples all over the globe consider Earth to be our mother. Look back at Chapter 1 and see how we literally must nurse from the earth and nature to obtain the minerals our

bodies need. Our culture, unfortunately, has lost this view, instead viewing the planet as an inanimate object to be exploited.
We think we can do better with our technology, our medicines,
and our fortified foods. As a society, we are now paying the
price for that disrespect of the earth through the widespread
functional mineral deficiencies, organic diseases, and the misery
these ailments create.

An Islamic sufi tradition says that in the time of Noah, the
people ridiculed him by throwing excrement into the ark, foul-
ing it. They then developed sores all over their bodies and
found that the only thing that would cure them was the excrement they had thrown at the ark. They scrubbed the ark clean
again to cure their sores. In a similar way, we as a people have
abused and disrespected the earth. But we get a better deal than
the people of Noah's time: We don't have to eat our pesticides,
garbage, and toxic waste to regain our health. We only need to
return to a diet rich in the earth's minerals.

The minerals in our body are like precious jewels, rare
gifts to us from the Creator. They perform biological functions
there that nothing can replace, not conventional or alternative
medical therapies, not mind/body medicine, not New Age
thinking. To maintain our health, or to regain a higher level of
health, we need only turn, open-handed, to receive the gift of
natural foods.

Where to Find a Practitioner of Nutritional Medicine

To find a physician who practices nutritional medicine, try the following referral resources.

American Association of Acupuncture and Oriental Medicine
433 Front St.
Catasauqua, PA 18032
(610) 433-2448

American Association of Naturopathic Physicians
601 Valley St., Suite 105
Seattle, WA 98109
(206) 298-0125 (referral line)

American College of Advancement in Medicine
P.O. Box 3427
Laguna Hills, CA 92654
(714) 583-7666

Canadian Association of Ayurvedic Medicine
P.O. Box 749, Station B
Ottawa, Ontario
Canada K1P 5P8

Price-Pottenger Nutrition Foundation
P.O. Box 2614
La Mesa, CA 91943
(619) 574-7763

PRODUCTS

SOURDOUGH BREADS MADE WITH SEA SALT

A-dough-B Bakery
113 West Park St.
Livingstone, MT 59047
(406) 222-3617

WHOLE ORGANIC GRAINS

Mountain Ark Traders
P.O. Box 3170
Fayetteville, AR 72702
(800) 643-8909

GRAIN MILLS

K-Tek
420 N. Geneva Road
Lindon, UT 84042
(801) 785-3600

UNREFINED OILS

Omega Nutrition
6505 Aldrich Road
Bellingham, WA 98226

Omega Nutrition's inventory includes coconut, walnut, flax, olive, and sunflower oils.

Sea Salt and Ionic Seawater Supplements

Grain and Salt Society
Box DD
Magalia, CA 95954
(916) 873-0294

Trace Minerals Research
P.O. Box 429
Roy, Utah 84067
(801) 731-6051

Seaweeds

Ryan Drum
Island Herbs
P.O. Box 25
Waldron Island, WA 98297

Maine Seaweed Company
P.O. Box 57
Stueben, ME 04680
(207) 546-2875

Wild Herbs

Frontier Herb Cooperative
P.O. Box 299
Norway, IA 52318
(800) 717-4372

Herb Seeds

Abundant Life Seed Foundation
P.O. Box 772
Port Townsend, WA 98368

Otto Richter and Sons
Goodwood
Ontario
Canada L0C 1A0

Books

Cholesterol and Health by Chris Mudd. American Lite Co., 1990.
Mudd reviews the dangers of a low-cholesterol, lowfat diet, with extensive scientific documentation.

Enzyme Nutrition by Dr. Edward Howell. Avery Publishing, 1986.
Describes the important role of food enzymes in raw foods and dairy products.

Lick the Sugar Habit by Nancy Appleton. Avery Press, 1996.
Appleton reviews the extensive scientific research on the adverse effects of sugar and presents a practical program for those who have sugar addictions.

Nourishing Traditions by Sally Fallon. ProMotion Publishing, 1995.
This book is a treasury of scientific information and recipes. Includes recipes from cultures around the world, with ways to prepare such traditional foods as organ meats, fermented grains and breads, and many more.

Nutrition and Physical Degeneration by Weston Price, D.D.S. Keats Publishing, 1938.
See Chapter 2 for a full discussion of this book.

Saccharine Disease: The Master Disease of Our Time by T. L. Cleave. Keats Publishing, 1975.
Cleave was one of the scientists who first scientifically documented the devastating effects of sugar as a regular component of the diet. This 1975 book is still in print.

Information Sources

The Price-Pottenger Nutrition Foundation
P.O. Box 2614
La Mesa, CA 91943
(619) 574-7763

The Price-Pottenger Nutrition Foundation was founded in the early 1960s to preserve the nutritional research of Dr. Weston Price and Dr. Francis Pottenger. The foundation is unique among nutrition research organizations in that it is completely free of government, medical, and industrial influences. It maintains a library; publishes a quarterly journal; maintains a referral list for nutritionally oriented doctors; and offers a number of excellent but hard-to-find books and videos for sale through a catalog. The library and book catalog preserve the works and research of a number of scientists whose nutrition research may otherwise have been forgotten, including:

> Dr. Francis Pottenger, who demonstrated the importance of raw foods in the diet.
>
> William Albrecht, Ph.D., who demonstrated the ill effects of soil depletion on animal and human nutrition.
>
> Dr. Edward Howell, who established the need for raw food enzymes in the diet and identified the dangers of enzyme inhibitors in some foods.
>
> John Myers, who demonstrated the value of ionic minerals for treating a wide variety of diseases.
>
> Dr. Melvin Page, who demonstrated the disturbing effects of sugar on the glandular system.

The Sea Greens Bulletin
Ted Spencer
P.O. Box 243
Crescent City, CA 95531
(707) 465-6335

Up-to-date research and other information on seaweeds.

REFERENCES

Abdulla, M., et al. 1975. "Dietary intake of potassium in the elderly." Letter. *Lancet* 2:562.

Abraham, A. S., et al. 1992. "The effects of chromium supplementation on serum glucose and lipids in patient with and without non-insulin dependent diabetes." *Metabolism* 41:768–771.

Abraham, G. 1992. "Management of fibromyalgia: Rationale for the use of magnesium and malic acid." *J. Nutr. Med.* 3:49–59.

Abrams, H. L. 1980. *Journal of Applied Nutrition* 32(2):70–71.

Adams, C. F. 1975. *Nutritive Value of American Foods in Common Units*. U.S. Department of Agriculture, Agriculture Handbook No. 456.

American Cancer Society. 1989. "Unproven methods of cancer treatment: Macrobiotic diets for the treatment of cancer." *CA: A Cancer Journal for Clinicians* 49:184–188.

American Cancer Society. 1993. "Questionable methods of cancer management: 'Nutritional' therapies." *CA: A Cancer Journal for Clinicians* 43:309–317.

Analytical Research Labs. Phoenix, Arizona. 1977.

Anderson, R. A., and Kozlovsky, A. S. 1985. "Chromium intake, absorption, and excretion of subjects consuming self-selected diets." *Am. J. Clin. Nutr.* 41:1177–1183.

Anderson, R. A., et al. 1987. "Effects of supplemental chromium on patients with symptoms of reactive hypoglycemia." *Metabolism* 36:351–355.

Anke, M., et al., eds. *Mengen-und Spurenelemente*. Leipzig: Arbeitstagung, 1981.

Appleton, N. *Lick the Sugar Habit*. Garden City Park, NY: Avery, 1997.

Arbman, G., et al. 1992. "Cereal Fiber, Calcium and Colorectal Cancer." *Cancer* 69:2042–2048.

Armstrong, P. L. 1989. "Iron deficiency in adolescents." *Br. Med. J.* 298:499.

Asai, Kazuhiko, Ph.D. *Miracle Cure: Organic Germanium*. Tokyo: Japan Publications Inc., 1980.

Aso, H., et al. 1989. "Antiviral activity of carboxyethylgermanium sesquioxide (Ge-132) in mice infected with influenza virus." *J. Biol. Response. Mod.* 8:180–189.

Basta, S. S., et al. 1979. "Iron deficiency anemia and the productivity of adult males in Indonesia." *Am. J. Clin. Nutr.* 32:6–25.

Beasley, J. *The Kellogg Report: The Impact of Nutrition, Environment, and Lifestyle on the Health of Americans.* Annandale-on-Hudson, NY: Institute of Health Policy and Practice, 1989.

Beasley, J. Lecture. Annual convention of the American Association of Naturopathic Physicians. Tempe, Arizona, 1992.

Behall, K., et al. 1987. "Mineral balance in adult men: effect of four refined fibers." *Am. J. Clin. Nutr.* 46:307–314.

Benfield, James W., D.D.S. July–September 1972. "Observations of Fluoridation of Public Water Supplies over a Period of 28 years." *National Fluoridation News* 2–3.

Bernstein, J., S. Alpert, K. Nauss, and R. Suskind. 1977. "Depression of lymphocyte transformation following glucose ingestion." *Am. J. Clin. Nutr.* 30:613.

Binder, T. Personal correspondence. August, 1996.

Birch, N. J., ed. *New Trends in Bio-inorganic Chemistry.* New York: Academic Press, 1978.

Block, G. 1979. "Dietary Guidelines and the results of food consumption surveys." *Am. J. Clin. Nutr.* 53:356S–357S.

Braunwald, E., K. J. Isselbacher, R. G. Petersdorf, J. D. Wilson, J. B. Martin, A. S. Fauci, eds. *Harrison's Internal Medicine.* 11th Ed. New York: McGraw-Hill, 1987.

Brennan, R. O. *Nutrigenics.* New York: M. Evans and Co., Inc., 1975.

Bricklin, M., ed. *The Natural Healing and Nutrition Annual.* Emmaus, PA: Rodale Press, 1989.

Bricklin, Mark. *The Practical Encyclopedia of Natural Healing.* New York: Penguin, 1990.

Burros, M. April 1, 1992. "No wonder doctors know little about nutrition." *New York Times.*

Bush, Irving, et al. Cook County Hospital, Chicago. "Zinc and the prostate." Presented at the annual meeting of the AMA, Chicago, 1974.

Cabrera, C. 1993. "The strange case of Mr. B." *Medical Herbalism* 5(4):1.

Canfield, W. "Chromium, glucose tolerance, and serum cholesterol in adults." In: Shapcott, D., and J. Hubert, eds. *Chromium in Nutrition and Metabolism.* New York: Elsevier, 1979.

Carl, E.G., et al. 1986. "Association of low blood manganese concentrations in epilepsy." *Neurology* 336:1584–1587.

Castelli, W. P. 1992. *Arch. Int. Med.* Cited in: Fallon.

Chandra, R. K. 1984. "Excessive intake of zinc impairs immune responses." *JAMA* 252(11):1443–1446.

Chapuy, M., et al. Dec. 3, 1992. "Vitamin D3 and Calcium to Prevent Hip Fractures in Elderly Women." *The New England Journal of Medicine* 327(23):1637–1642.

Cohen, A. 1963. *American Hebrew Journal* 65:291. Cited in: Fallon.

Cohen, N., et al. 1996. "Oral vanadyl sulfate improves insulin sensitivity in NIDDM but not in obese nondiabetic subjects." *Diabetes* 45(5):659–666.

Coleman, D. C., E. P. Odum, and D. A. Crossley, Jr. 1992. "Soil biology, soil ecology and global change." *Biol. Fert. Soils* 14:104–111.

Colgan, M. *Your Personal Vitamin Profile.* New York: William Morrow, 1982.

Contempre, B., et al. 1992. "Effects of selenium supplementation on thyroid hormone metabolism in an iodine and selenium deficient population." *Clin. Endocrinology* 36:579–583.

Constantini, A. V. et al. June 1997. "The fungal/mycotoxin etiology of atherosclerosis and hyperlipidemia." *Townsend Letter for Doctors* #197.

Constantinidis, J. 1991. "The Hypothesis of Zinc Deficiency in the Pathogenesis of Neurofibrillary Tangles." *Med. Hypo.* 35:319–323.

Constantinidis, J. 1992. "Treatment of Alzheimer's Disease by Zinc Compounds." *Drug Development Research* 27:1–14.

Dale, G., et al. 1987. "Fitness, unfitness and phosphate." *British Medical Journal* 294:939.

Dean, C. *Dr. Carolyn Dean's Complementary Natural Prescriptions for Common Ailments.* New Canaan, CT: Keats Publishing, Inc., 1994.

Donaldson, J., and A. Barbeau. "Manganese neurotoxicity: Possible clues to the etiology of human brain disorders." In: Gabay, S., et al, eds. *Metal Ions in Neurology and Psychiatry.* New York: Alan R. Hiss, 1985. pp. 259–285.

Donahue, R. L. *Our Soils and Their Management* Danville, IL: Interstate, 1970.

Dreno, B., et al. 1989. "Low Doses of Zinc Gluconate for Inflammatory Acne." *ACTA Der. Vener Stockh.* 69:541–543.

Drum, R. *Seaweeds for Therapy.* P.O. Box 25, Waldron Island, WA 98297.

Ebeling, W. *The Fruited Plain: The Story of American Agriculture.* Berkeley, CA: University of California Press, 1979.

Eby, G. A., et al. 1984. "Reduction in duration of common colds by zinc gluconate lozenges in a double blind study." *Antimicrob. Agents Chemother.* 25:20–24.

Ensminger, A. H., M. E. Ensminger, J. F. Konlande, and J. R. K. Robson. *Food and Nutrition Encyclopedia.* Clovis, CA: Pegus Press, 1983.

Erasmus, U. *Fats That Heal, Fats That Kill.* Burnaby, B.C.: Alive Books, 1993.

Eskin, B. A., et al. 1967. "Mammary gland dysplasia in iodine deficiency." *AMA* 200:115.

Evans, G. W., et al. 1993. "Composition and biological activity of chromium-pyridine carbosylate complexes." *J. Inorganic Biochemistry* 49:177–187.

Fallon, S. *Nourishing Traditions*. San Diego: ProMotion Publishing, 1995.

Franz, K. B. 1987. "Magnesium intake during pregnancy." *Magnesium*. 6:18–27.

Freeland-Graves, J. H., Ph.D., R.D. November/December 1988. "Manganese: An Essential Nutrient for Humans." *Nutrition Today* pp. 13–19.

Frieden, E., ed. *Biochemistry of the Elements*. New York: Plenum, 1984.

Ganapathy, S., and R. Dhanda. 1980. "Protein and iron nutrition in lacto-ovo-vegetarian Indo-Aryan United States residents." *Indian J. Nutr. Diet* 17:45-52.

Garland, C., et al. 1985. "Dietary Vitamin D and Calcium and the Risk of Colorectal Cancer: A 19 year Prospective Study in Men." *Lancet* 1:307–309.

Garland, C., and F. Garland. *The Calcium Connection*. New York: G. P. Putnam's Sons, 1988.

Giller, R. M., and Kathy Matthews. *Natural Prescriptions*. New York: Carol Southern Books, 1994.

Gittleman, A. L. *Beyond Pritikin*. New York: Bantam, 1980.

Gordenoff, T., and W. Member. 1962. "Fluorine." *World Review of Nutrition and Dietetics* 2:213.

Gordon, A. M. October 1992, "Effects of Adjunctive Therapy with Zinc in Human Immunodeficiency Virus Infection." Journal of the American College of Nutrition 11(5):601, Abstract No. 17.

Goredeuk, V., et al. 1987. "Iron overload: causes and consequences." *Ann. Nutr. Rev.* 7:485–508.

Griffith, H. W. *Complete Guide to Vitamins, Minerals and Supplements*. Tuscon, AZ: Fisher Books, 1988.

Griffiths, Norman. Feb. 22, 1990. "New Rap Against Fluoride: P&G Study." *Medical Tribune*.

Guiness, A. E., ed. *The ABC's of the Human Body*. Pleasantville, N.Y.: The Reader's Digest Association, Inc., 1987.

Hall, R. H. *Food for Thought: The Decline in Nutrition*. New York: Harper and Row, 1974; New York: Random House/Vintage Books, 1976.

Halliday, J., and L. Powell. "Iron overload." *Sem. Hematol.* 1982:19:42-53

Hamaker, J. *The Survival of Civilization*. Burlingame, CA: Hamaker-Weaver Publications, 1982.

Hambridge, K. M., et al. 1983. "Zinc nutritional status during pregnancy: a longitudinal study." *Am. J. Clin. Nutr.* 37:429–442.

Harland, B. F., and B. A. Harden-William. 1993. "Is vanadium of human nutritional importance yet?" *J. Am. Diet. Assoc.* 94:891–894.

Harris, R. S. "Effects of agricultural practices on the Composition of Foods, Part 1." In: Harris R. S., and E. Karmas, eds. *Nutritional Evaluation of Food Processing*, 2nd Ed. Westport, CT, 1975.

Hendler, S. S., M.D. *The Doctor's Vitamin and Mineral Encyclopedia*. New York: Simon & Schuster, 1990.

Hendrix, P. F., R. W. Parmelee, D. A. Crossley, Jr., D. C. Coleman, E. P. Odum, and P. M. Groffman. 1986. "Detritus foodwebs in conventional and no-tillage agroecosystems." *Bioscience* 36:374–380.

Herring, M. Jan. 29, 1986. "Calcium Supplements May Prove Hedge Against Colon Cancer." *Medical Tribune*.

Hocman G. 1988. "Chemoprevention of Cancer: Selenium." *Int. J. Biochem.* 20:123–132.

Hornick, S. B. 1992. "Factors affecting the nutritional quality of crops." *Am. J. Alt. Ag.* 7(1 and 2).

Ingham, R. E., J. A. Trofymow, E. R. Ingham, and D. C. Coleman. 1985. "Interactions of bacteria, fungi, and their nematode grazers: Effects on nutrient cycling and plant growth." *Ecol. Monogr.* 55:119–140.

Ingham, R. E. "Interactions between invertebrates and fungi: Effects on nutrient availability," pp. 669–690. In: G. C. Carroll and D. T. Wicklow, eds. *The Fungal Community: Its Organization and Role in the Ecosystem*, 2nd Ed. New York: Marcel Dekker, 1992.

Jenkins, G. N. "Molybdenum." In: *Trace Elements and Dental Disease*. Curzon, M. E. J., and T. W. Cutress, eds. Boston: John Wright, 1983.

Jiang He et al. March 1991. "Relationship of Electrolytes to Blood Pressure in Men: The Xi Peoples Study." *Hypertension* 17(3):378–385.

Journal of the American Medical Association. 1982. 248(12):1465. Cited in: Fallon.

Kariks, J. 1988. "Cardiac lesions in sudden infant death syndrome." *Forensic Sci. Int.* 39:211–215.

Katts et al. 1991. "The effects of chromium picolinate supplementation on body composition in different age groups: Age 14." Abstract No. 40.

Kidd, Pariss M., Ph.D. January 1987. "Germanium-132 (Ge-132) Homeostatic Normalizer and Immunostimulant. A Review of Its Preventative and Therapeutic Efficacy." International Clinical Nutrition Review 7(1):11–19.

Kies, C., et al. "Zinc bioavailability from vegetarian diets: Influence of dietary fiber, ascorbic acid, and past dietary practices." In: Inglett, G. E., ed. *Nutritional Bioavailability of Zinc*. ACS Series No. 210. Washington, D.C.: American Chemical Society, 1983.

Kirchfeld, F., and W. Boyle. *The Nature Doctors*. Portland: Medicina Biologica, 1994.

Kiremidjian-Schumacher, L., and G. Stotsky. 1987. "Selenium and immune responses." *Environmental Res.* 42:277–303.

Kiremidjian-Schumacher, L., et al. 1994. "Supplementation with selenium and human immune cell functions; II Effect on cytotoxic lymphocytes and natural killer cells." *Biol. Trace Elem. Res.* 41:115–127.

Koop. E. *The Surgeon General's Report on Nutrition and Health.* Washington, D.C.: USGPO, 1988.

Korpela, H., et al. 1989. "Effect of selenium supplementation after acute myocardial infarction." *Res. Commun Chem. Pathol. Pharmacol.* 65:249–252.

Krause, M. V., and K. L. Mahan. *Food Nutrition and Diet Therapy.* 7th Ed. Philadelphia: W. B. Saunders, 1984.

Krouse, T. B., et al. 1979. "Age Related Changes Resembling Fibrocystic Breast Disease in Iodine Blocked Rats." *Arch. Pathol. Lab. Med.* 103:631–634.

Kumpulainen, J. T. 1979. "Determination of chromium in selected U.S. diets." *J. Agric. Food. Chem.* 27(3):490–494.

Lassus, A. 1993. "Colloidal silicic acid for oral and topical treatment of aged skin, fragile hair and brittle nails in females." *J. Int. Med. Res.* 21:209–215.

Lee, T. C., and G. O. Chichester. "The Influence of Harvest Time on Nutritional Value." In: White, P.L., and N. Selvey, eds. *Nutritional Qualities of Fresh Fruits and Vegetables.* Mount Kisco, NY: Futura Publishing, 1974.

Lemke, R., and A. Schafer et al. 1993. "Postmortem serum selenium concentrations and their possible etiological role in sudden infant death (SID)." *Forensic Sci. Int.* 60:179–182.

Lenihan, J. *The Crumbs of Creation: Trace Elements in History, Medicine, Industry, Crime, and Folklore.* New York: Adam Hilger, 1988.

Levin, B. 1992. "Nutrition and Colorectal Cancer." *Cancer* 70(6):1723–1726, Suppl.

Lindlahr, H. *Natural Therapeutics: Vol III, Dietetics.* Saffron Walden, England: C. W. Daniel Company, 1914 (reprinted with commentary, 1983).

Longnecker et al. *Nutrition and Cancer Prevention: Investigating the Role of Micronutrients.* New York: Marcel Dekker, 1989.

Losee, F. L., and B. L. Adkins. 1969. "A study of the mineral environment of caries-resistant navy recruits." *Caries Res.* 3:23–31.

Lozoff, B., M.D. Sept 5, 1991. "Long term developmental outcome of infants with iron deficiency." *New England Journal of Medicine* 325: 687–694.

Luo, X. M., and H. J. Wei et al. 1983. "Inhibitory effect of molybdenum on esophageal and forestomach cancer." *National Cancer Institute Journal* 71:75–80.

MacDonald, A., Ph.D, R.D. *The Complete Book of Vitamins and Minerals.* Lincolnwood, IL: Publications International, Ltd., 1996.

Malhotra, S. 1968. *Indian Journal of Industrial Medicine* 14:219. Cited in: Fallon.

Marsh, A. G, et al. 1980. "Cortical bone density of adult lacto-ovo-vegetarian and omnivorous women." *J. Am. Dietetic Assn.* 76:148–151.

Marsh, A. G., et al. 1983. "Bone mineral mass in adult lacto-ovo-vegetarian and omnivorous males." *Am. J. Clin. Nutr.* 37:453–456.

Marttineau, J., et al. 1985. "Vitamin B$_6$, Magnesium, and Combined B$_6$ Magnesium Therapeutic Effects in Childhood Autism." *Biol. Psychiat.* 20:467–478.

Marz, R. *Medical Nutrition from Marz*. Portland: Omnivites Press, 1997.

Matsusaka, T., et al. 1988. "Germanium induced nephropathy: Report of two cases and review of the literature." *Clinical Nephrology* 30:341–345.

Maugh, T. H. 1978. "The fatted calf (II): The concrete truth about beef." *Science* 199, Jan. 27.

McDougall, J. *McDougall's Medicine: A Challenging Second Opinion*. Piscataway, NJ: New Century Publishers, Inc., 1985.

McNeill, J. H. June 16, 1993. "Biological Effects of Vanadium." The University of British Columbia, B.C.

Meredith, T. J., and J. A. Vale. January 1987. "Treatment of paraquat poisoning in man: Methods to prevent absorption." *Hum. Toxicol.* 6(1):49–55.

Mertz, W. 1993. "Chromium in human nutrition: A review." *J. Nutr.* 123:626–633.

Michelson, D., et al. 1996. "Bone mineral density in women with depression." *New England Journal of Medicine* 335(16):1176–1181.

"Molybdenum deficiency in TPN." 1987. *Nutr. Rev.* 45(11):337–341.

Money, D. F. L. 1970. "Vitamin E and selenium deficiencies and their possible etiological role in the sudden infant death syndrome." *NZ Med. J.* 71:32–34.

Mooradian, A. D., et al. 1987 "Micronutrient status in diabetes mellitus." *Am. J. Clin. Nutr.* 45:877–895.

Morgan, K. J., et al. 1985. "Magnesium and calcium dietary intakes of the U.S. population." *J. Am. Coll. Nutr.* 4:195.

Murphy, E. J., E. Roberts, and L. A. Horrocks. 1993a. "Aluminum silicate toxicity in cell cultures." *Neuroscience* 55(2):597–605.

Murphy, E. J., E. Roberts, D. K. Anderson, and L. A. Horrocks. 1993b. "Cytotoxicity of aluminum silicates in primary neuronal cultures." *Neuroscience* 57(2):483–490.

Murray, F. *The Big Family Guide to All the Minerals*. New Canaan, CT: Keats Publishing, 1995.

Murray, M., N.D. *Encyclopedia of Nutritional Supplements*. Rocklin, CA: Prima Publishing, 1996.

National Academy of Sciences. *Nutrition Education in Medical Schools.* National Academy Press, 1985.

National Center for Toxicological Research, U.S. Food and Drug Administration. Noted in: *FDA Consumer.* May 1991.

NIH Consensus Conference: Osteoporosis. 1984. *JAMA* 252(6):799–802.

Netter, A., et al. 1981. "Effect of zinc administration on plasma testosterone, dihydrotestosterone and sperm count." *Arch. Androl.* 7:69–73.

Newsome, D. A. 1988. "Oral Zinc in Macular Degeneration." *Archives of Ophthalmology* 106:192–198.

Nielsen, F. H. September 1996 . "How should dietary guidance be given for mineral elements with beneficial actions or suspected of being essential?" *J. Nutr.* 126(9 Suppl):2377S–2385S.

Neilsen, F. H. "Vanadium." In: Mertz, W., ed. *Trace Elements in Human and Animal Nutrition,* Vol. 1. New York: Academic Press, 1987.

Nielsen, F. H., et al. 1987. "Effect of dietary boron on mineral, estrogen, and testosterone metabolism in postmenopausal women." *FASEB J.* 1:394–397.

1987 Curriculum Directory of the Association of American Medical Colleges. Medical school hours are averages of Johns Hopkins, Mayo, Yale, and Stanford medical schools.

Nolan, K. B. 1983. *Nutr. Rev.* 41:318–320.

"Nutrient Deficiency Causing Mass Ills." December 16, 1994. *The Tennessean.*

Odeh, M. 1992. "The role of Zinc in Acquired Immunodeficiency Syndrome." *Journal of Internal Medicine* 231:463–469.

O'Keeffe, S. T., K. Gaavin, and J. N. Lavan. 1994. "Iron Status and Restless Leg Syndrome in the Elderly." *Aging* 23:200–203.

Olmsted, L., and G. N. Schrauzer et al. 1989. "Selenium Supplementation of Symptomatic Human Immunodeficiency Virus Infected Patients." *Bio. Trace Elem. Research.* 20:59.

Ouchi, Y., et al. 1991. "Effects of Dietary Magnesium on Development of Atherosclerosis on Cholesterol Fed Rabbits." *Biology and Trace Elements* 30:59–64.

Papavasiliou, P., et al. 1979. "Seizure disorders and trace metals: Manganese in epileptics." *Neurology* 29:1466–1473.

Parley, Dixie. October 1986. "The Buildup and Breakdown of Bone Tissue." *FDA Consumer* p. 34.

Pfeiffer, C. C., S. and LaMola. 1983. "Zinc and manganese in the schizophrenias." *J. Orthomolecular Psychiatry* 12:215–234.

Pfeiffer, C. C., Ph.D., M.D. *Nutrition and Mental Illness.* Rochester, VT: Healing Arts Press, 1987.

Pizzorno, J. *Total Wellness*. Rocklin, CA: Prima Publishing, 1996.

Prasad, A. S. 1991. "Role of zinc in human health." *Contemp. Nutr.* 16(5).

Press, R. I., et al. 1990. "The effect of chromium picolinate on serum cholesterol and apolipoprotein fractions in human subjects." *Western Journal of Medicine* 152:41–45.

Price, W. A. 1914. "Some contributions to dental and medical science." *Dental Summary* 34:253.

Price, W. A. *Dental Infections, Oral and Systemic*. Cleveland, OH: Penton, 1923.

Price, W. A. *Nutrition and Physical Degeneration*. New Canaan, CT: Keats Publishing, 1938.

Reid, I. R., et al. 1995. "Long-term effects of calcium supplementation on bone loss and fractures in post menopausal women: A randomized controlled trial." *Am. J. Med.* 98:331–335.

Riggs, B., et al. 1990. "A four year controlled trial of fluoride supplementation of women with osteoporosis does not change fracture rate." *New England Journal of Medicine* 332:802.

Rimland, B. 1988. "Controversies in the Treatment of Autistic Children: Vitamin and Drug Therapy." *J. Child Nev.* 3:568–572.

Ringsdorf, W., E. Cheraskin, and R. Ramsay. 1976. "Sucrose, neutrophilic phagocytosis and resistance to disease." *Dent Surv* 52:46–48

Rose, G., et al. 1983. *Lancet* 1:1062–1065. Cited in: Fallon.

Rouse D. J., et al. 1996. "The feasibility of a randomized clinical perinatal trial: Maternal magnesium sulfate for the prevention of cerebral palsy." *Am. J. Obstet. Gynecol.* 175:701–705.

Roy, M. 1994. "Supplementation with selenium and human immune cell functions; I Effect on lymphocyte proliferation and interleukin 2 receptor expression." *Biol. Trace Elem. Res.* 41:103–114.

Rubinstein A. H., N. W. Levin et al. 1962. "Manganese induced hypoglycemia." *Lancet* 2:1348–1351.

Safai-Kutti, S. 1990. "Oral Zinc Supplementation in Anorexia Nervosa." *ACTA Psychiatr. Scand.* 361(82):14–17 Suppl.

Samuels, A. J. 1965. "Studies in patients with functional menorrhagia: The anti-hemorrhagic effect of the adequate repletion of iron stores." *Israel J. Med. Sci.* 1:851.

Sanchez, A., J. Reese, H. Lau, et al. 1973. "Role of sugars in human neutrophilic phagocytosis." *Am. J. Clin. Nutr.* 26:1180–1184.

Sanstead, H. H. 1973. *Am. J. Clin. Nutr.* 26:1251–1260.

Sardesai, V. M. 1993. "Molybdenum: An essential trace element." *Nutr. Clin. Pract.* 8:277–281.

Sato, I., and B. D. Yuan et al. 1985. "Inhibition of tumor growth and metastasis in association with modification of immune response by novel organic germanium compounds." *J. Biol. Response. Mod.* 4:159–168.

Schauss, A. G. 1991. "Nephrotoxicity in humans by the ultratrace element germanium." *Ren. Fail.* 13(1):1–4.

Schauss A. G. , Ph.D. *Minerals, Trace Elements, and Human Health.* Tacoma, WA: Life Sciences Press, 1995.

Schechter, Michael, M.D., et al. November 1992. "Rationale of Magnesium Supplementation in Acute Myocardial Infarction, a Review of the Literature." *Archives of Internal Medicine* 152: 2189–2196.

Schell T. C., M. D. Lindemann, E. T. Kornegay, D. J. Blodgett, and J. A. Doerr. May 1993. "Effectiveness of different types of clay for reducing the detrimental effects of aflatoxin-contaminated diets on performance and serum profiles of weanling pigs." *J. Anim. Sci.* 71(5):1226–31.

Schoenmann, H. M., et al. 1990. "Consequences of severe copper deficiency are independent of dietary carbohydrate in young pigs." *Am. J. Clin. Nutr.* 52:147–154.

Scholl, T., et al. 1992. "Anemia vs. Iron Deficiency: Increased Risk of Preterm Delivery in a Prospective Study." *Am. J. Clin. Nutr.* 55:985–988.

Schrauzer, G. N., and K. P. Shrestha et al. 1992. Biol. Trace Elem. Res. 34:161–170.

Schroeder, H. A. 1968. "The role of chromium in mammalian nutrition." *Am. J. Clin. Nutr.* 21(3):230–244.

Schwarz, K. 1977. "Silicon, fiber and atherosclerosis." *Lancet* 1:454–456.

Scott, C. *Crude Black Molasses.* New York: Benedict Lust Publications, 1980.

Seelig, M. *Magnesium Deficiency in the Pathogenesis of Disease.* New York: Plenum Press, 1980.

Seggev, M. "International Osteoporosis Experts Convene in the United States." Recap of the Research Advances in Osteoporosis conference, Washington, D.C., February 26, 1990.

"Selenium deficiency, thyroid hormone metabolism and thyroid hormone deiodinases." 1993. *Am. J. Clin. Nutr.* 57:236S–248S.

Shaker, J. L., K. W. Krawczyc, and J. W. Finding. 1986. "Primary hyperparathyroidism and severe hyperclacemia with low circulating 1,25-dihydrooxyvitamin D levels." *J. Clin. Endocrinol. Metab.* 62:1305–1308.

Shils, M. E., and V. R. Young. *Modern Nutrition in Health and Disease.* 7th Ed. Philadelphia: Delea and Kebiger, 1988.

Simkin, P. A. 1976. "Oral Zinc Sulphate in Rheumatoid Arthritis." *Lancet* 2:539–542.

Simopaulus, A. P., and N. Salem. 1992. *Am. J. Clin. Nutr.* 55:411–414.

Singh, A., et al. 1989. "Magnesium, zinc, and copper status of U.S. Navy SEAL trainees." *Am. J. Clin. Nutr.* 49:695–700.

Smith, B. L. 1993. "Organic foods vs. supermarket foods: Element levels." *J. Appl. Nutr.* 45(1):35–38.

Soskel, N. T., et al. 1982. "A copper deficient, zinc supplemented diet produces emphysema in pigs." American Review of Respiratory Disease. 126:316.

Spak, C.-J., et al. 1989. "Tissue response of gastric mucosa after ingestion of fluoride." *Br. Med. J.* 298;1686–1687.

Stadel, B. V. April 24, 1976. "Dietary Iodine and Risk of Breast, Endometrial and Ovarian Cancer." *Lancet.*

Stewart, R. E. "Technology of Agriculture," *Encyclopedia Britannica* 15th Ed, 1977.

Stone, W. L., M.D. *Annals of Nutrition and Metabolism.* 1986.

Surawicz, B., et al. 1957. "Clinical manifestations of hypopotassemia." *Am. J. Med. Sci.* 233:603.

Suzuki, F., and R. R. Brutkiewicz, et al. 1986. "Cooperation of lymphokines and macrophages in expression of antitumor activity of carboyethlgermanium sesquioxide." *Anticancer Res.* 6:177–182.

Tanzi, R., M.D., quoted in "Experiments Link Alzheimer's Condition to Zinc." Sept. 6, 1994. *New York Times.*

Taymor, M. L., S. H. Sturgia, and C. Yahia. 1964. "The etiological role of chronic iron deficiency in menorrhagia." *JAMA* 187:323.

Thoma, K., and H. Lieb. 1983. "Absorption of drug substances by antacids and adsorbents and their influence on bioavailability." *Dtsch. Apoth. Ztg.* 123(24):2309–2316.

Tortora, G. *Introduction to the Human Body.* 3rd Ed. New York: Biological Sciences Textbooks, Inc., 1994.

Touitou, Y., et al. 1987. "Prevalence of magnesium and potassium deficiencies in the elderly." *Clin. Chem.* 33:518–523.

Unsworth, E. F., J. Pearce, C. H. McMurray, B. W. Moss, F. J. Gordon, and D. Rice. September 1989. "Investigations of the use of clay minerals and prussian blue in reducing the transfer of dietary radiocaesium to milk." *Sci. Total Environ.* 85:339–47.

U.S. Bureau of the Census. *Statistical Abstract of the U.S.: 1996* (116th Ed.) Washington, D.C., 1996.

U.S. Department of Agriculture, Agricultural Research Service. *Composition of Foods; Raw, Processed, Prepared.* Agriculture Handbook No. 8. 1963 (reprinted in 1975).

U.S. Department of Agriculture, Agricultural Research Service. *Composition of Foods: Poultry Products; Raw, Processed, Prepared.* Agriculture Handbook No. 8–5. 1979.

U.S. Department of Agriculture, Agricultural Research Service. *Composition of Foods: Fruits and Fruit Juices; Raw, Processed, Prepared.* Agriculture Handbook No. 8–9, 1982.

U.S. Department of Agriculture, Agricultural Research Service. *Composition of Foods: Vegetables and Vegetable Products; Raw, Processed, Prepared.* Agriculture Handbook No. 8–11, 1984.

U.S. Department of Agriculture, Agricultural Research Service. *Composition of Foods: Nut and Seed Products; Raw, Processed, Prepared.* Agriculture Handbook No. 8–12, 1984.

U.S. Department of Agriculture, Agricultural Research Service. *Composition of Foods: Finfish and Shellfish Products; Raw, Processed, Prepared.* Agriculture Handbook No. 8–15, 1987.

U.S. Department of Agriculture, Agricultural Research Service. *Composition of Foods: Legumes and Legume Products; Raw, Processed, Prepared.* Agriculture Handbook No. 8–16, 1986.

U.S. Department of Agriculture, Agricultural Research Service. *Composition of Foods: Fast Foods; Raw, Processed, Prepared.* Agriculture Handbook No. 8–21, 1988.

U.S. Department of Agriculture, Agricultural Research Service. *Composition of Foods: Lamb, Veal, and Game Products; Raw, Processed, Prepared.* Agriculture Handbook No. 8–17, 1989.

U.S. Department of Agriculture, Agricultural Research Service. *Composition of Foods: Cereal Grains and Pasta; Raw, Processed, Prepared.* Agriculture Handbook No. 8–20, 1989.

U.S. Department of Agriculture, Agricultural Research Service. *Composition of Foods: Beef Products; Raw, Processed, Prepared.* Agriculture Handbook No. 8–13, 1990.

U.S. Department of Agriculture, Agricultural Research Service. *Composition of Foods: Raw, Processed, Prepared.* Agriculture Handbook No. 8. 1989 Supplement, 1990; 1990 Supplement, 1991; 1991 Supplement, 1992a; 1992 Supplement, 1993.

U.S. Department of Agriculture, Agricultural Research Service. *Composition of Foods: Pork Products; Raw, Processed, Prepared.* Agriculture Handbook No. 8–10, 1992b.

U.S. Department of Agriculture, Agricultural Research Service. *Composition of Foods: Baked Products; Raw, Processed, Prepared.* Agriculture Handbook No. 8–18, 1992c.

U.S. Department of Agriculture. 1992d. "Food and Nutrient Intakes by Individuals in the United States, 1 Day, 1989–91," NFS Rep. No. 91–2.

U.S. Department of Agriculture, Economic Research Service. *Food Consumption, Prices, and Expenditures, 1996: Annual Data, 1970–1994.* Statistical Bulletin No. 928, April 1, 1996.

U.S. Department of Agriculture, Agricultural Research Service. Nutrient Database SR11, 1997.

U.S. Department of Agriculture, Food Surveys Research Group. Results from the 1994 CSFII. www.barc.usda.gov/bhnrc/foodsurvey/home.htm, 1997b.

Viteri, F. E., and B. Torun. 1974. "Anemia and physical work capacity." *Clin. Haematol.* 3:609–626.

Voors, A. W., M.S., Shuman, and Gallagher. 1971. *World Rev. Nutr. Diet* 20:299–326.

Walker, W. R., and D. M. Keats. 1976. "An investigation of the therapeutic value of the copper bracelet—dermal assimilation of copper in arthritic/rheumatoid conditions." *Agents and Actions* 6:454–458.

Wallach, J. D., and M. Lan. *Rare Earths: Forbidden Cures.* Bonita, CA: Double Happiness Publishing Company, 1994.

Wasowicz, W. 1994. "Selenium concentration and glutathione peroxidase activity in blood of children with cancer." *J. Trace. Elem. Electrolytes Health. Dis.* 8:53057.

Webster, P. O. 1987. "Magnesium." *Am. J. Clin. Nutr.* 45(5 Suppl):1305–1312.

Weinberg, E. D. 1984. "Iron withholding: A defense against infection and neoplasia." *Physiol. Rev.* 64:65–102.

Whittaker, C. W., et al. 1959. "Liming qualities of three cement kiln flue dusts and a limestone in a greenhouse comparison." Soil and Water Cons. Res. Div., USDA, Beltsville, MD.

Whittaker, C. W., et al. 1963. "Cement kiln flue dusts for soil liming." U.S. Fertilizer Lab, Soil and Water Cons. Res. Div., USDA, Beltsville, MD.

Wolfe, S. M., R.-E. Hope. *Worst Pills, Best Pills II.* Washington, D.C.: Public Citizen's Health Research Group, 1993.

Worthington-Roberts, B. "Suboptimal nutrition and behavior in children." *Contemporary Developments in Nutrition.* St. Louis: 1981.

INDEX